INSULIN RESISTANCE DIET 2025

100 Healthy Recipes Advanced Nutritional Strategies for Optimal Health Meal Plans and Tips for Stabilizing Blood Glucose

KLARLOCK

DISCLAIMER

This book aims to provide useful and informative material on the topics covered in the publication. It is sold with the understanding that the author and publisher are not engaged in rendering any personal medical, health care, or other professional services in the book. The reader should consult his or her physician, health care provider, or other competent professional before adopting any suggestions in this book or drawing any conclusions. The author and publisher expressly disclaim any responsibility for any liability, loss, or risk, personal or otherwise, arising, directly or indirectly, from the use and application of any contents of this book.

NOTE

All the recipes in this book are designed for four people. For this quantity, the ingredients indicated in the recipes must be considered. If you need to change the portion, it is recommended to proportionally adjust the doses of the ingredients. It is also recommended to carefully follow the preparation and cooking instructions to obtain the best result. In the context of this book, when we refer to "a cup" as a unit of measurement for ingredients, we mean using a standard kitchen cup with a capacity of approximately 240 milliliters. It is essential to use a measuring cup to get the right quantities of ingredients. If you don't have a measuring cup, you can use a graduated measuring cup, making sure to correctly correspond to the proportions indicated. Here are some examples 1 Cup of flour 100 gr. 1 cup of rice 200 gr. 1 Cup of Quinoa 200 gr

TABLE OF CONTENT

RECIPES FIRST DISHES

RECIPES SECOND DISHES

INTRODUCTION INSULIN RESISTANCE

Insulin resistance is a condition in which the body's cells become less sensitive to insulin, a hormone produced by the pancreas that regulates blood sugar levels. When cells do not respond adequately to insulin, the body tries to compensate by producing more insulin. This can lead to high blood sugar levels and, over time, can contribute to the development of type 2 diabetes and other metabolic complications. Importance of Diet in Managing Insulin Resistance One of the most effective strategies for managing insulin resistance is through diet. Choosing appropriate foods can improve insulin sensitivity, help maintain stable blood sugar levels, and prevent complications.

A vegetarian diet, in particular, can be very beneficial due to its high content of fiber, antioxidants and essential nutrients, as well as reducing the consumption of saturated fats which can aggravate insulin resistance. Book Objectives This book aims to: 1. Educate readers about insulin resistance, its causes, symptoms, and long-term consequences. 2. Provide detailed guidance on how a well-balanced vegetarian diet can help manage and improve insulin resistance. 3. Offer practical advice, recipes and food plans to facilitate the adoption of a healthy and sustainable lifestyle. 4. Motivate readers to make informed food choices to improve their overall health and prevent chronic diseases related to insulin resistance.

UNDERSTANDING INSULIN RESISTANCE

Definition and causes of insulin resistance Insulin resistance is a metabolic condition in which the cells of the body, mainly the muscles, liver and adipose tissue, become less sensitive to the action of insulin. Insulin is a hormone essential for the metabolism of carbohydrates, fats and proteins. The causes of insulin resistance are multifactorial and include: 1. Genetics: Genetic predisposition can play a significant role in the development of insulin resistance. 2. Obesity: Excess body fat, especially visceral, is strongly associated with insulin resistance. 3. Sedentary lifestyle: Lack of physical activity reduces the sensitivity of cells to insulin. 4. Poor diet: A diet rich in refined sugars,

Saturated fat and low fiber contributes to the development of insulin resistance. 5. Stress: Chronic stress and its hormonal effects can negatively affect insulin sensitivity. 6. Sleep disorders: Insufficient or poor-quality sleep is associated with an increased risk of insulin resistance. Symptoms and diagnosis Insulin resistance can be asymptomatic for many years. However, some signs and symptoms may indicate the presence of this condition: 1. Increased hunger: Constant feeling of hunger despite food intake. 2. Weight gain: Particularly in the abdominal area. 3. Fatigue: Persistent feeling of tiredness. 4. Difficulty concentrating: Mental confusion or difficulty maintaining attention. 5. Darkening of the skin: Acanthosis nigricans, characterized by areas of dark, thickened skin, often on the neck or under the armpits.

To diagnose insulin resistance, doctors may use several tests: 1. Measuring fasting blood sugar: Elevated fasting blood sugar levels may indicate insulin resistance. 2. Oral Glucose Tolerance Test (OGTT): Measures the body's response to a glucose load. 3. Fasting insulin levels: Elevated fasting insulin levels may indicate insulin resistance. 4. HOMAIR Index: Calculated using fasting blood glucose and insulin values, it provides an indication of insulin sensitivity.

NUTRITIONAL PRINCIPLES BALANCING OF MACRONUTRIENTS

A balanced nutritional approach is essential to manage insulin resistance. Here's how macronutrients—carbs, proteins, and fats—need to be balanced to support insulin sensitivity and keep blood sugar levels stable. 1. Carbohydrates Carbohydrates are the main source of energy for the body, but it is important to choose the right ones to avoid glycemic spikes. Complex Carbohydrates: Whole Grains: Oats, quinoa, spelled, brown rice. Legumes: Lentils, chickpeas, beans. Vegetables: Particularly non-starchy ones such as spinach, broccoli, cauliflower. Simple Carbohydrates: Limit: Refined sugars, sugary drinks, sweets and industrial baked goods. Fruit: Prefer whole fruit to fruit juices for the fiber content. Glycemic Index (GI): Prefer Low GI Foods: Foods that release glucose slowly into the blood, keeping sugar levels stable. Examples of Low GI Foods: Barley, lentils, apples, pears. 2. Proteins Proteins are essential for growth, tissue repair and maintenance of muscle mass. Sources of Lean Protein: White Meat: Chicken, skinless turkey. Fish: Particularly rich in omega3 fatty acids such as salmon, mackerel, sardines. Eggs: Complete source of protein and other nutrients. Legumes: Beans, lentils, peas. Low Fat Dairy Products: Greek yogurt, ricotta, skim milk. Vegetable Proteins: Tofu, tempeh, seitan, nuts and seeds. Recommended Amounts: Adequate Portion: Approximately 20/30% of daily calories should come from proteins, based on individual needs and level of physical activity.

3. Fats Fats are crucial for hormonal health and the absorption of fat-soluble vitamins. However, not all fats are created equal. Healthy Fats: Monounsaturated Fats: Olive oil, avocado, nuts, seeds. Polyunsaturated Fats: Fish oil, flax seeds, chia seeds. Omega3 Fatty Acids: Essential for reducing inflammation and improving insulin sensitivity. Saturated and Trans Fats: Limit: Saturated fats (found in red meat, butter, cheese) and avoid trans fats (found in industrial baked goods and fried foods). Recommended Quantities: Adequate Portion: Approximately 25/35% of daily calories should come from fats, favoring unsaturated ones. 4. Fiber Fiber is essential for good digestion and for keeping blood sugar levels stable. Soluble Fiber: Sources: Oats, apples, carrots, citrus fruits. – Benefits: They slow down the absorption of glucose and improve insulin sensitivity. Insoluble Fibers: Sources: Cereals

wholemeal, nuts, green leafy vegetables. Benefits: Improve intestinal health and prevent constipation. Recommended intake: Quantity: Approximately 25/30 grams per day for women and 30/38 grams per day for men. Meal Planning Example Breakfast: Oat porridge with fresh fruit and nuts. Lunch: Quinoa salad with chickpeas, avocado, spinach and tomatoes. Grilled salmon fillet with broccoli and brown rice. Dinner: Peppers stuffed with ground turkey and vegetables. Tofu stir fry with mixed vegetables and brown rice. Snack: Carrot sticks with hummus. Apple with almond butter. Balancing macronutrients appropriately can significantly improve the management of insulin resistance, helping to maintain stable blood sugar levels and promoting optimal health.

BENEFITS OF THE INSULIN RESISTANCE DIET

Adopting a diet specifically for insulin resistance can lead to numerous health benefits. Here are some of the main benefits that people can get: Improved Insulin Sensitivity 1. Reduced Resistance: A balanced diet can reduce insulin resistance by making it easier to transport glucose into cells and keeping blood sugar levels below check. 2. Stabilization of Glucose Levels: Avoiding glycemic spikes helps keep blood sugar levels stable, preventing symptoms such as tiredness, irritability and sudden hunger. Weight Loss and Weight Control 1. Reduction of Visceral Fat: A diet high in fiber and low in refined carbohydrates can help reduce visceral fat, which is closely linked to insulin resistance.

2. Increased Satiety: Foods rich in fiber and protein can increase feelings of satiety, reducing overall calorie intake and facilitating weight loss. Improved Cardiovascular Health 1. Reduce Cholesterol and Triglycerides: Low glycemic index foods and healthy fats can reduce LDL (bad) cholesterol and triglyceride levels, improving heart health. 2. Regulation of Blood Pressure: A balanced, nutrient-rich diet can help keep blood pressure within normal limits. Prevention of Type 2 Diabetes 1. Risk Reduction: Managing insulin resistance with an appropriate diet can significantly reduce the risk of developing type 2 diabetes. 2. Prediabetes Management: For those who are prediabetic, a targeted diet can reverse the condition and prevent progression to diabetes.

Improved Energy and General Wellbeing 1. Increased Energy: Avoiding blood sugar spikes and maintaining stable blood sugar levels leads to a steady increase in energy levels. 2. Improved Mental Wellbeing: A balanced diet can improve mood, reduce stress and increase mental clarity. Improved Digestive Function 1. Increase Fiber Intake: A diet rich in fiber promotes intestinal health, improving digestion and preventing constipation. 2. Gut Flora Balance: Probiotic and prebiotic foods help maintain a healthy gut microbiome, which is linked to metabolic health. Immune System Support 1. Essential Nutrients: A diet rich in vitamins, minerals and antioxidants can strengthen the immune system, protecting the body from diseases.

2. Reduce Inflammation: Anti-inflammatory foods can reduce chronic inflammation, which is a risk factor for many chronic diseases. Longevity and Quality of Life 1. Increased Longevity: A healthy and balanced diet can contribute to a longer and healthier life, reducing the risk of chronic diseases. 2. Improved Quality of Life: Effectively managing insulin resistance improves quality of life, allowing people to live more active and satisfying lives.

CONCLUSION AND FUTURE OF THE DIET

Final Reflection The journey towards managing insulin resistance through diet is a journey of awareness, education and sustainable lifestyle changes. Understanding the importance of balancing macronutrients, choosing low glycemic index foods, integrating physical activity and adopting healthy habits are key steps to improving insulin sensitivity and preventing long-term complications. Key Takeaways from the Book: Understanding Insulin Resistance: Definition, Causes, Symptoms, and Health Implications. Nutritional Principles: Balance of macronutrients, importance of fibre, choice of foods with a low glycemic index. Examples of Meal Plans: Practical ideas for balanced and nutritious meals. Role of Physical Activity:

Types of recommended exercises and their benefits. Healthy Lifestyle: Stress management, sleep quality and other healthy habits. Testimonials: Success stories of people who have improved their situation. Looking to the Future Diet Evolution for Insulin Resistance: Research and Innovation: The science of nutrition is constantly evolving. New research may provide further information on how to improve the management of insulin resistance. Personalization: Personalized diets based on genetic analyzes and individual biomarkers may become increasingly accessible and widespread. Technology and Apps: The use of apps for monitoring diet, glucose level and physical activity can offer continuous and personalized support. Tips for the Long Term: Continuing Education: Stay up to date on the latest research and nutritional advice to adapt and improve your diet.

RECIPES APPETIZERS

BRUSCHETTA WITH TOMATO AND BASIL

Preparation time: 10 minutes

Cooking time: 15 minutes

Doses for 2 people:

Ingredients:

4 slices of stale bread

2 ripe tomatoes, cut into cubes

1/2 red onion, finely chopped

1 clove garlic, finely chopped

2 tablespoons extra virgin olive oil

1 tablespoon balsamic vinegar

10 fresh basil leaves, chopped

Salt to taste

Freshly ground black pepper to taste

Preparation:

Preheat the oven to 180°C. Arrange the slices of stale bread on a baking tray. In a large bowl, combine the diced tomatoes, the finely chopped red onion, the finely chopped garlic, the extra virgin olive oil, the balsamic vinegar, the chopped fresh basil, a pinch of salt and a grind of black pepper. Mix everything well and spread the tomato mixture on each slice of bread. Bake in the oven for about 15 minutes, or until the bruschettas are golden and crispy. Remove the bruschetta from the oven and serve immediately.

Nutritional values (per serving):

Calories: 250 kcal

Fat: 12 g

Protein: 6 g

Carbohydrates: 30 g

CHICKPEA HUMMUS WITH CRISPY VEGETABLES

Preparation time: 15 minutes

Cooking time: 1 hour

(if using dried chickpeas)

Doses for 2 people:

Ingredients:

200 g of dried chickpeas

(or 400g canned chickpeas)

1 clove of garlic

1/2 lemon juice

2 tablespoons tahini

2 tablespoons extra virgin olive oil

1/4 teaspoon cumin powder

Salt to taste

Freshly ground black pepper to taste

Raw vegetables to accompany

(e.g. carrots, celery, peppers)

Preparation:

If using dried chickpeas, rinse them and soak them in cold water for at least 8 hours. Cook the chickpeas in boiling water for about 1 hour, or until tender. Drain the chickpeas and rinse them under running water. In a food processor or blender, combine the cooked chickpeas, garlic, lemon juice, tahini, extra virgin olive oil, cumin powder, a pinch of salt and a grind of black pepper . Blend everything until you obtain a smooth and creamy mixture. If necessary, add a little water to thin the hummus. Transfer the hummus into a bowl and serve with the raw vegetables cut into sticks. Nutritional values (per serving):

Calories: 350 kcal Fat: 15 g

Protein: 18 g Carbohydrates: 40 g

QUINOA AND AVOCADO SALAD

Preparation time: 15 minutes

Cooking time: 15 minutes

Doses for 2 people:

Ingredients:

1 cup rinsed quinoa

2 cups of water

1 ripe avocado, cut into cubes

1/2 cup cherry tomatoes, cut in half

1/4 cup cucumber, diced

1/4 cup crumbled feta

2 tablespoons black olives, pitted and cut into slices

2 tablespoons extra virgin olive oil

1 tablespoon lemon juice

1/2 teaspoon dried oregano

Salt to taste

Freshly ground black pepper to taste

Preparation:

Rinse the quinoa under running water to remove the saponin. In a medium saucepan, combine the rinsed quinoa and water. Bring to the boil, then reduce the heat, cover and cook for 15 minutes, or until the quinoa has absorbed all the liquid and the sprouts are visible. Remove the pan from the heat and let the quinoa rest for 5 minutes with the lid still closed. Fluff the quinoa with a fork to separate the grains. In a large bowl, combine the cooked quinoa, diced avocado, halved cherry tomatoes, diced cucumber, crumbled feta and sliced black olives.

Season with extra virgin olive oil, lemon juice, dried oregano, salt and freshly ground black pepper. Mix everything well and serve immediately. Nutritional values (per serving):

Calories: 450 kcal (approximately)

Fat: 20 g

Protein: 18 g

Carbohydrates: 50 g

CAPRESE WITH BUFFALO MOZZARELLA AND TOMATOES

Preparation time: 10 minutes

Cooking time: 0 minutes

Doses for 2 people:

Ingredients:

250 g of fresh buffalo mozzarella

500 g of cherry tomatoes

Fresh basil

Extra virgin olive oil

Salt to taste

Freshly ground black pepper to taste

Preparation:

Wash the cherry tomatoes and cut them into slices. Cut the buffalo mozzarella into slices. Arrange the cherry tomatoes and buffalo mozzarella in layers on a serving plate. Garnish with fresh basil leaves. Season with extra virgin olive oil, a pinch of salt and a grind of black pepper. For a more intense flavour, you can use perfectly ripe seasonal cherry tomatoes. You can also add other ingredients to the salad, such as olives, capers or oregano. Serve immediately.

Nutritional values (per serving):

Calories: 400 kcal (approximately)

Fat: 25 g

Protein: 25 g

Carbohydrates: 30 g

BAKED ZUCCHINI FRITTERS

Preparation time: 20 minutes

Cooking time: 20/25 minutes

Doses for 2 people:

Ingredients:

2 medium courgettes, grated

50 g of 00 flour

2 eggs

50 g of grated parmesan

50 ml of milk

1 clove garlic, finely chopped

1 sprig of fresh parsley, chopped

Salt to taste

Freshly ground black pepper to taste

Extra virgin olive oil for greasing

Preparation:

Preheat the oven to 180°C. In a large bowl, combine the grated courgettes, flour, eggs, grated parmesan, milk, chopped garlic, chopped parsley, a pinch of salt and a grind of black pepper. Mix everything well until you obtain a homogeneous mixture. Line a baking tray with baking paper and grease it with a drizzle of extra virgin olive oil. Using a spoon, form small pancakes with the courgette mixture and place them on the baking tray. Bake in the oven for about 20-25 minutes, or until the pancakes are golden and crispy. Remove the courgette fritters from the oven and serve them hot.

Nutritional values (per serving):

Calories: 250 kcal (approximately)

Fat: 15 g

Protein: 10 g

Carbohydrates: 25 g

SALMON AND AVOCADO TARTARE

Preparation time: 15 minutes

Cooking time: 0 minutes

Doses for 2 people:

Ingredients:

200 g of fresh chilled salmon,

stripped of skin and thorns

1 ripe avocado

1/2 red onion, finely chopped

1 tablespoon lemon juice

1 tablespoon extra virgin olive oil

Salt to taste

Freshly ground black pepper to taste

Capers for garnish (optional)

Preparation:

With a sharp knife, finely chop the fresh salmon. In a large bowl, combine the chopped salmon, the diced avocado, the finely chopped red onion, the lemon juice, the extra virgin olive oil, a pinch of salt and a grind of black pepper. Mix everything well with a spoon until you obtain a homogeneous mixture. Serve the salmon and avocado tartare on a bed of green salad or on croutons. Garnish with capers (optional).

Nutritional values (per serving):

Calories: 400 kcal (approximately)

Fat: 30 g

Protein: 25 g

Carbohydrates: 5 g

MELON AND HAM SKEWERS

Preparation time: 10 minutes

Cooking time: 0 minutes

Doses for 4 people:

Ingredients:

500 g of melon

200 g of raw ham

10 fresh mint leaves

Salt to taste

Freshly ground black pepper to taste

Preparation:

Cut the melon into cubes of about 2 cm. Fold the slices of raw ham in half. Thread a cube of melon, a slice of raw ham folded in half and a mint leaf onto a skewer. Repeat the process until the skewers are complete. Season with a pinch of salt and a grind of black pepper. Serve the melon and raw ham skewers cold.

Nutritional values (per serving):

Calories: 200 kcal (approximately)

Fat: 10 g

Protein: 15 g

Carbohydrates: 20 g

POLENTA CROSTINI WITH MUSHROOMS

45

Preparation time: 20 minutes

Cooking time: 30 minutes

Doses for 4 people:

Ingredients:

300 g of corn flour for polenta

1 liter of water

Salt to taste

300 g of mixed mushrooms

1 clove garlic, finely chopped

2 tablespoons extra virgin olive oil

Preparation:

In a large pot, bring salted water to a boil. Pour in the corn flour and mix with a whisk to avoid lumps. Cook the polenta for about 30 minutes, stirring occasionally, until the mixture is thick and creamy. Pour the polenta onto a wooden cutting board and spread it with a damp spoon to a thickness of about 1 cm. Leave the polenta to cool completely. Cut the polenta into squares and lightly grill them on a non-stick pan. In a pan, heat the extra virgin olive oil and fry the chopped garlic for a minute.

Add the sliced mixed mushrooms and cook for about 10 minutes, or until tender. Salt and pepper to taste. Arrange the mushrooms on the polenta croutons and serve.

Advice

For a more intense flavor, you can use porcini mushrooms or other wild mushrooms. You can also add other ingredients to the mushroom salad, such as olives, cherry tomatoes or peppers.

Nutritional values (per serving):

Calories: 350 kcal (approximately)

Fat: 15 g

Protein: 10 g

Carbohydrates: 45 g

COURGETTE CARPACCIO WITH PARMESAN

Preparation time: 15 minutes

Cooking time: 0 minutes

Doses for 2 people:

Ingredients:

2 medium courgettes

100 g of parmesan

Fresh basil

Extra virgin olive oil

Salt to taste

Freshly ground black pepper to taste

Preparation:

Wash the courgettes and dry them with a clean cloth. Using a mandolin or slicer, cut the courgettes into thin slices like a carpaccio. Arrange the courgette slices on a serving plate. Cut the parmesan into flakes with a potato peeler. Spread the parmesan flakes over the courgettes. Garnish with fresh basil leaves. Season with a drizzle of extra virgin olive oil, a pinch of salt and a grind of black pepper. Serve the courgette carpaccio with parmesan immediately.

Nutritional values (per serving):

Calories: 150 kcal (approximately)

Fat: 10 g

Protein: 5 g

Carbohydrates: 10 g

AUBERGINES ROLLS WITH RICOTTA AND WALNUTS

Preparation time: 30 minutes

Cooking time: 45 minutes

Doses for 4 people:

Ingredients:

2 medium aubergines

250 g of ricotta

50 g chopped walnuts

50 g of grated parmesan

1 egg

Fresh basil

Extra virgin olive oil

Salt to taste

Freshly ground black pepper to taste

Preparation:

Wash the aubergines and cut them into slices
lengthwise, approximately 1 cm thick. Grill
the aubergine slices on a hot grill for about 5
minutes per side, or until soft. In a large
bowl, combine the ricotta, chopped walnuts,
grated Parmigiano Reggiano, egg, a pinch of
salt and ground black pepper. Mix
everything well until you obtain a
homogeneous mixture. Spread the ricotta
mixture over each slice of grilled aubergine.
Roll the aubergine slices on themselves to
form rolls. Arrange the aubergine rolls on a
baking tray. Season with a drizzle of extra
virgin olive oil and garnish with fresh basil
leaves.

Bake in a preheated oven at 180°C for about 20 minutes, or until the rolls are golden. Remove the aubergine rolls with ricotta and walnuts from the oven and serve them hot or warm.

Advice:

For a more intense flavour, you can also add some grated pecorino cheese to the ricotta mixture. You can also use chopped walnuts to decorate the rolls before serving them.

Nutritional values (per serving):

Calories: 350 kcal (approximately)

Fat: 20 g

Protein: 20 g

Carbohydrates: 30 g

RECIPES
FIRST DISHES

GREEN APPLE RISOTTO

Time 50 min

ingredients

4 servings

360 g of Carnaroli rice

a shallot

an organic Granny Smith apple

Lemon

sugar

dry white wine

mint leaves

vegetable broth

extra virgin olive oil

salt, black pepper

Preparation

For the green apple risotto recipe, peel the apple, keeping the peel, and divide it into 6 segments. Cook it in a pan with water acidulated with the juice of half a lemon for 1520 minutes, then drain it well and blend the apple. Cut the apple peels into very thin strips. Bring 2 tablespoons of water to the boil with 2 tablespoons of sugar; turn off, let cool, immerse the apple peels, mix well and leave to rest. Peel and chop the shallot. Fry it in a pan with a drizzle of oil, then add a spoonful of broth and let it simmer for 2 minutes, stirring. Toast the rice in an anti-grease pan for about 3 minutes, then pour in half a glass of very cold wine;

When the wine has evaporated, cover the rice thinly with the boiling broth, add the shallot and a spoonful of oil and continue cooking for 15 minutes, adding a ladle of broth from time to time. When the rice is cooked and dry, add the apple puree and mix vigorously until blended. Season with salt and season with a drizzle of raw oil. Distribute the risotto onto plates and garnish with apple peels in syrup, a few mint leaves and a generous grind of black pepper.

SPRING MINESTRONE

Time 40 min

ingredients

68 servings

350 g of courgettes

350 g of new potatoes

250 g of red cherry tomatoes

150 g of green beans

150 g of yellow carrots

100 g snow peas

100 g of celery

100 g of carrots

marten, thyme, mint

vegetable broth, salt

Preparation

For the spring minestrone recipe, blanch the cherry tomatoes in boiling salted water for a minute, then remove the peel and cut them in half. Clean all the vegetables and cut them into small pieces. Cook the potatoes in the vegetable broth for 3 minutes, then add the carrots; after 2 minutes add the celery and after another 2 minutes the green beans, snow peas and courgettes; cook everything together for another 10 minutes; finally complete with the cherry tomatoes and cook for another 2 minutes. Turn off the heat and add marjoram, thyme and mint leaves in equal quantities. Season with salt, season with a drizzle of raw oil and serve.

TUSCANY STYLE TOMATO PAPPA

Time 1h 30min

ingredients

4 servings

1 kg of ripe tomato pulp

200 g of Tuscan bread

3 cloves of garlic

basil

extra virgin olive oil

salt

Pepper

Preparation

For the tomato soup recipe, fry the chopped garlic and a nice sprig of basil in oil until they start to sizzle. Add the tomato pulp crushed with a fork and season with salt and pepper. Cook over moderate heat for about 20'. Add the sliced bread, cover everything with hot water and leave to infuse for a few minutes, then turn off the heat and leave to rest, covered, for an hour. Before serving, stir vigorously to break up the bread and, if necessary, heat the gelatine.

VEGETARIAN RISOTTO

Time 40 min

ingredients

6 servings

360 grams of rice

180 g of courgettes

150 g of carrots

150 mg of dry white wine

60 g grated parmesan

60 g onion, peeled

40 grams of butter

before Belgian endive

1 L of broth (also stock cube)

olive oil, salt

Preparation

For the vegetarian risotto recipe, trim, trim and wash the escarole. Drain it and cut it into strips. Clean the courgettes and carrots; scrape the latter then cut both vegetables into cubes. Chop the onion and sauté it in 2 tablespoons of oil, then add the vegetables and lightly salt. When everything is wilted, add the rice, raise the heat and toast it. Then add the wine and, after this has evaporated, lower the heat and continue cooking the risotto, stirring often and adding the hot broth little by little. Turn off when the rice is slightly al dente and still wavy and stir in the butter and parmesan. Cover and let rest for a couple of minutes before serving the risotto on a suitable plate.

CAULIFLOWER WITH ORANGE E BLACK RADISH SAUCE

Time 1h

ingredients

4 people

500 g of green cauliflower

200 g black radish

1 medium golden apple

1 orange

sugar, salt

extra virgin olive oil

apple cider vinegar

Preparation

For the cauliflower with orange and radish sauce recipe, peel the radishes and apple and finely grate. Collect in a bowl and season them with 1 tablespoon of apple cider vinegar and 2 tablespoons of oil, 1 teaspoon of sugar and one of salt. Clean the cauliflower by removing the thicker leaves. Cook it in boiling salted water with the orange peel, juice and the rest of the citrus fruits. After 15/20 minutes, drain it and keep the orange and its peel aside. Spray a baking tray, lined with baking paper, with 5 tablespoons of oil, place the cauliflower, and season with salt and 2 tablespoons of oil. To keep the cauliflower standing, use the slices and orange peel. Cook at 200°C for 15 minutes on the highest shelf of the oven; continue with the grill mode for 5/7 minutes, until a golden crust forms. Serve hot with the sauce. Cauliflower can be kept in the fridge for 3 days and is also good cold, in a salad. perhaps reinforced with tuna in oil and olives.

VEGETARIAN LASAGNA

Time 1h 40min

ingredients

Servings for 6 people

For the vegetable sauce

600 g of fresh pasta for lasagne

400 g of tomatoes

300 g of lentils

300 grams of leek

100 g of carrots

2 shallots

fresh chili pepper, thyme

dry white wine

Rosemary

extra virgin olive oil

vegetable broth, salt and pepper

Complete

1 liter of bechamel

pecorino cheese

extra virgin olive oil

Preparation

For the vegetable sauce, soak the lentils in cold water for 1 hour. Peel and chop the carrots, leeks and shallots. Prepare an aromatic bunch with thyme, rosemary and 1/2 fresh chilli pepper. Cut the tomatoes with a cross cut and blanch them for 1 minute; remove the skin and cut them into small pieces.

Fry the chopped vegetables in a saucepan with 4 tablespoons of oil for 34 minutes; add the lentils, blend with 1 glass of wine, add the bouquet garni, mix and cook for another 34 minutes; add the chopped tomatoes, cook for 5 minutes, then add a ladle of broth, salt, pepper and cook for another 16/18 minutes. To complete, compose the lasagna with the "ragù" and the béchamel, finishing with a layer of lentils, strips of pecorino and a drizzle of oil; cook in a fan oven at 190°C for 15 minutes.

RISOTTO WITH PEAS

Time 25 min

ingredients

1 serving

200 g of vegetable broth

60 g of Carnaroli rice

30 g of shelled peas

20 g of red onion

2 teaspoons extra

virgin olive oil

parsley

Preparation

To prepare the risotto with peas, heat the vegetable broth. Finely chop the onion, brown it in the oil without letting it brown, add the shelled peas, let them flavor for a minute, then add a spoonful of hot broth. Cook them for 5 minutes, then add the rice and continue cooking with the remaining boiling broth. The risotto will be ready after about 15/18 minutes and must be very soft. Serve immediately, completing with a pinch of chopped parsley. You can also use frozen peas: in this case add the rice and peas to the onion at the same time.

PAKCHOI TO TE EASTERN

Time 30 min

ingredients

4 servings

150 g tamari sauce

30 g of lemon juice

20 g mirina

8 g of corn starch

2 pakchoi

Lemon

sugar

Rosemary

extra virgin olive oil

sesame

Preparation

For the oriental pakchoi recipe, divide the pakchoi in half lengthwise, cut off the base and blanch in boiling water for 23 minutes, keeping the leaves out of the water. Drain them, combine them well with the oil and grill for 2 minutes per side. Bring the tamari sauce to the boil with 50 g of water, lemon juice and mirin. Dilute the cornstarch with a little water and add it to the sauce, with a teaspoon of sugar and a pinch of finely grated lemon zest. Continue cooking for 12 minutes, stirring. Toast 3 tablespoons of sesame seeds in a pan and distribute them on the pakchoi, together with rosemary leaves. Serve the sauce separately.

BAKED PUMPKIN WITH CABBAGE AND HAZELNUTS

Time 1h

ingredients

4 people

850 g of organic pumpkin

300 g whole cabbage leaves

50 g of hazelnuts

1 small golden onion

extra virgin olive oil

sugar

Rosemary

White wine

salt and pepper

Preparation

For the baked pumpkin with cabbage and hazelnuts recipe, crush one part of the hazelnuts with the flat blade of the knife to break them in half, leaving the other whole. Toast them in the oven at 200°C for 5 minutes. Clean the pumpkin from the seeds and the internal beard but leave the zest; cut it into slices about 5 mm thick. Clean the onion, removing the heads but leaving it seasoned with a layer of peel; cut it into wedges. Place the pumpkin on a baking tray covered with baking paper and drizzle with 4 tablespoons of oil. Make sure the slices don't overlap. Peel the onion segments and arrange the leaves here and there in the pan. Season everything with 4 tablespoons of oil, 2 pinches of salt and rosemary sprigs and bake at 200°C for 30 minutes. Blanch the whole cabbage leaves in boiling salted water for 34 minutes, taking care to keep them under water (help yourself with a ladle if necessary). Then drain them and cool them in very cold water. Drain them very well and arrange them slightly overlapping on a baking tray covered with baking paper and lightly greased. Drizzle the cabbage with 3 tablespoons of oil and 3 tablespoons of white wine, add a pinch of salt and a pinch of sugar and cook in the oven at 200°C for about 10 minutes. Serve the pumpkin hot on the cabbage, sprinkle with hazelnuts and complete with pepper. The zest is very tasty and can be eaten (if the pumpkin is organic).

COLD VEGETARIAN TIMBALLO

Time 1h 50min

ingredients

6 people

Zuchinis

130 g of yellow courgettes

130 g of green courgettes

130 g of trumpet courgettes

130 g of Roman-style courgettes

salt, extra virgin olive oil

The pasta

1 kg of tomatoes, 500 g of bucatini

250 g of stracciatelle

50 g of pitted black olives

40 g of desalted capers

½ spring onion, dried oregano

extra virgin olive oil, fennel

sugar, basil, salt and pepper

Preparation

For the courgettes, peel all the courgettes and cut them into 34 mm thick slices. Sprinkle a large pan with a little salt, arrange a layer of courgette slices and cook for 23 minutes so that they remain crunchy. Repeat until the courgettes are finished (they must not overlap during cooking). Place them in a baking dish, season them with 60/100 g of oil and let them cool. For the pasta, cut the cherry tomatoes into 4 segments, remove the seeds and place them on a baking tray lined with baking paper; season generously with oil, salt, sugar and dried oregano. Bake at 160°C for about 40 minutes. Collect capers, olives and plenty of coarsely chopped herbs (fennel, basil, oregano) in a bowl and season with 30 g of oil. Remove the tomatoes from the oven and blend with 1/2 spring onion, season with salt and pepper and pour into the bowl with the capers and olives. Boil the pasta and drain it al dente, add it to the sauce in the bowl and mix carefully. Line a courgette mold (ø 20 cm, h 10 cm) with transparent film, and cover the entire internal surface of the mold with the courgette slices, making them adhere well to the film. Place half the pasta in the mold, add the stracciatella, cover with the rest of the pasta, press lightly and close the bottom with cling film; put in the fridge for 45 hours. Remove from the fridge, remove the film from the bottom, turn out onto a serving plate, remove the film and serve the timbale cold, decorating as desired with capers and aromatic herbs.

CAPPELLETTI DI ROMAGNA WITH CLAMS AND SPINACH

Time 1h 30min + 9h rest

ingredients

6 people

For Cappelletti

300 g of 00 flour

150 g of fresh ricotta

150 g of soft cheese

30 g grated parmesan

3 eggs, salt and pepper

nutmeg, parsley

For the sauce

1 kg clams

150 g of tomato puree

50 g of new spinach

2 copper tomatoes

dry white wine

extra virgin olive oil

garlic, salt, pepper

Preparation

For the Cappelletti, form a fountain with the flour on a wooden surface, place the eggs in the center and beat with a fork, scooping the flour by hand until it is all incorporated; then work with your hands until you obtain a smooth, soft and homogeneous dough. Cover it with cling film and let it rest for 30/60 minutes at room temperature. Mix the ricotta and any other soft, fresh cheese in a bowl, with a little finely chopped parsley, parmesan and a little nutmeg. Adjust the filling with salt and pepper. Roll out the dough thin (12 mm) with a rolling pin or with the appropriate machine, cut out discs (ø 67 cm), place 1 teaspoon of filling in the center of each disc, and close by first sealing the overlapping edges and then joining the corners forming the classic shape of a hat. Soak the clams in lightly salted water for 5 hours (store them in the least cold part of the refrigerator). Then rinse and clean them. Heat 3 tablespoons of oil and 1 clove of garlic in a fairly large pan over high heat. When the garlic is a little coloured, add the clams, blend with a little (less than 1/2 glass) of white wine and cover with a lid to let the clams open; once opened, remove them from the pan with their sauce and remove the garlic.

Pour 2 tablespoons of oil into the same pan, heat 1 clean clove of garlic over a high heat, then add the tomato puree, reduce to a medium heat; when it boils, add the tomato pulp cut into cubes. Add all the liquid clam sauce again and leave to cook for 5/10 minutes over high heat. Shell the clams and add them to the tomato in the pan. Cook for another 2 minutes. Blend the spinach with an immersion blender, with 2 tablespoons of oil, a pinch of salt and freshly ground pepper. Keep aside. Cook the cappelletti in boiling salted water until they float to the surface. Drain them and let them flavor in the pan with the sauce for 2 minutes. Serve hot, complete with a few drops of spinach pesto.

SPAGHETTI WITH SAFFRON, SEA URCHIN CRISPY QUINOA

Time 1h

ingredients

4 people

360 grams of spaghetti

50 g of puffed quinoa

4 sea urchins

1 clove of garlic

saffron

anchovy sauce, lemon

fish soup, sunflower seed oil

extra virgin olive oil

salt and pepper

Preparation

For the recipe for spaghetti with saffron, sea urchins and crunchy quinoa, toast 30 g of saffron pistils in a saucepan with a pinch of salt and a drizzle of oil. Pour in 2 liters of fish broth, bring to the boil and cook for about 10 minutes. Turn off, let rest for 15 minutes, then filter and let cool. Brown the garlic in a large pan with a drizzle of oil and salt for 2 minutes. Remove the garlic, add the saffron broth and let it reduce. Cook the spaghetti in boiling salted water. Drain them al dente and pour them into the pan with the saffron sauce. Mix the pasta with oil, salt, pepper and drops of anchovy sauce. Fry the quinoa in sunflower oil. Serve the spaghetti with the puffed quinoa and the cleaned sea urchins; complete with grated lemon zest.

SPAGHETTI WITH PORCINI AND PECORINO

Time 25 min

ingredients

4 servings

350 grams of spaghetti

100 g of pecorino

4 porcini mushroom caps

extra virgin olive oil

salt

pepper in grains

Preparation

For the spaghetti with pecorino recipe, heat the water in a large pan and, when it boils, add salt and add the spaghetti. In the meantime, clean the caps of the porcini mushrooms and cut them into slices. In a pan, dry toast some ground pepper, add a drizzle of oil, the porcini mushrooms and sauté for 2 minutes; then pour in 1 ladle of pasta cooking water and cook for another 1 minute. Collect the pecorino in a bowl and mix it with 1 ladle of pasta water to create a sauce. Drain the spaghetti al dente directly into the pan with the mushrooms and add a little more water to complete cooking. Remove from the heat, add the pecorino sauce, mix well and serve.

VALPELLINESE SOUP

Time 1h

ingredients

4 people servings

600 grams of cabbage

400 g of meat broth

400 g of rye bread

300 g Fontina cheese

150 grams of butter

100 grams of lard

1 egg, salt, pepper

Preparation

For the Zuppa alla Valpellinese recipe, blend the bread with the fontina cheese with the food processor. Also add the egg, salt and pepper and mix until you obtain a homogeneous mixture.

Form these into balls, as big as olives. Clean the cabbage and cut it into strips, keeping 2 whole leaves aside for decoration. Melt 100 g of butter in a saucepan together with the lard. When they have melted, add the strips of cabbage and let them flavour, stirring; close with the lid and leave to cook for about 56 minutes. Then add the broth and cook for another 20 minutes. In the meantime, brown the bread and cheese balls in a pan with 50 g of butter for about 56 minutes. Add them to the cabbage casserole and cook everything together for another 10/12 minutes. Toast the cabbage leaves kept aside in the microwave: spread them on the tray and cook in the microwave at maximum power for 78 minutes, for 30 seconds at a time, turning the leaves at each interval.

LASAGNA WITH AUTUMN VEGETABLES

Time 1h 10min

ingredients

6 people

1 liter bechamel

500 g of flour

200 g of cleaned pumpkin

200 g of cleaned celeriac

200 g of carrots

5 eggs

Grated Parmesan cheese

extra virgin olive oil

salt and pepper

Preparation

For the lasagna recipe with autumn vegetables, mix the flour and eggs in the planetary mixer. Let the dough rest covered for 30 minutes. Using the vegetable chopper, slice the pumpkin and celeriac and grate the carrots. Fry the vegetables with oil, salt and pepper. Roll out the dough with the sheeter to 1 mm. Compose the lasagna by alternating the pasta with bechamel, vegetables and parmesan. Bake at 180°C for about 20 minutes. Serve hot.

TAGLIOLINI WITH POTATOES BACON AND COD

Time 1h 15 min +

2h marination

ingredients

4 people

For the cod

200 g desalted cod

thyme, marjoram

parsley, oregano

salty, tarragon

extra virgin olive oil

For Tagliolini

400 g of flour

6 egg yolks

extra virgin olive oil, salt

For Potato Cream

400 g of vegetable broth, 300 g of potatoes

40 g of extra virgin olive oil

To complete, 200 g of bacon

extra virgin olive oil

oregano (or parsley)

Preparation

For the cod, remove the skin and bones from the cod and cut it into cubes. Collect them in a baking dish, season them with a drizzle of oil, then add all the sprigs of aromatic herbs. Cover with cling film and leave to marinate in the fridge for 2 hours. For the Tagliolini Mix the flour with the egg yolks, 1 tablespoon of oil, approximately 100 g of water and a pinch of salt: mix everything together until you obtain a smooth and elastic dough, wrap it in cling film and let it rest in the refrigerator for at least 30 minutes. For the potato cream, peel the potatoes, cut them into chunks and boil them in the broth for 15/20 minutes. Blend everything, slowly adding the oil. Season with salt. To complete, roll out the pasta into very thin sheets, using a pasta machine, then cut it to obtain tagliolini. Cut the bacon into pieces and brown them in a pan with a drizzle of oil for 2 minutes, until they start to become crispy. Boil the tagliolini in boiling salted water for 1 minute and drain them with a ladle directly into the pan with the bacon: sauté them briefly with the little cooking water they brought with them.

ADMIRAL'S SOUP

Time 30 min

ingredients

4 people

1 liter vegetable broth

240 g of boiled chickpeas

230 g of swordfish

150 grams of rice

60 g of almonds in their skin

50 g of white vinegar, 40 g of raisins

20 g of candied citron

15 g of sugar, 4 biscuits

1 sachet of saffron

half an onion, salt

extra virgin olive oil

Preparation

For the Admiral's Soup recipe, chop the onion and brown it in a saucepan with a drizzle of oil for 23 minutes. Add the rice and toast it for 2 minutes, then add the broth and saffron. Cook for about 25 minutes, adding the chickpeas in the last 5 minutes. Bring the vinegar and sugar to the boil and cook for 20 minutes, until reduced to a syrup. Cut the candied citron into cubes and soak the raisins in water. Cut the swordfish into chunks and brown it for 12 minutes in a pan with oil and salt. Season it with citron, raisins and vinegar syrup. Place on the biscuits and serve them together with the soup, completing with the chopped almonds.

RAVIOLI WITH CHICORY WITH CHESTNUT CREAM

Time 2h 30min

ingredients

8 servings

For the pasta, 250 g of flour

125 g of egg yolks, salt

For the stuffing

250 g of red radicchio

250 g of ricotta

40 g of mature cheese

1 pc shallot, salt and pepper

extra virgin olive oil

Complete

200 g of fresh chestnuts

100 g of sliced bacon, sage, salt

Preparation

For the ravioli, For the recipe for radicchio ravioli with chestnut cream, beat the egg yolks with 20 g of water. Place the flour on the work surface forming a fountain and pour the beaten egg yolks and a pinch of salt into the center. Start kneading the egg yolks and flour with a fork, then knead by hand, gather the dough into a ball, wrap it in cling film and leave it to rest in the fridge for 1 hour. For the filling, peel the radicchio and cut it into slices. Fry it in a pan with a drizzle of oil and the chopped shallot for 3 minutes, stirring constantly, then mixed with the ricotta, the coarsely chopped cheese, salt and pepper. To complete the pasta in long sheets 12 mm thick.

Stuff half with the walnuts in the filling, cover them with other sheets of pasta, making them adhere well around the filling; cut about sixty square ravioli. Boil the chestnuts and peel them; Blend 100 g into a cream with 80 g of boiling water and a little salt. Brown the bacon in a large non-stick pan with a few sage leaves until it becomes crispy. Season 30 g of boiled chestnuts in the same pan as the bacon. Boil the ravioli in plenty of boiling salted water; once they come to the surface, drain them and add them to the pan with the chestnuts with a couple of spoons of their cooking water; let them flavor off the heat. Arrange them on plates with the chestnut cream, bacon and sage and serve immediately.

SPINACH VELVETE

Time 30 min

ingredients

6 servings

650 g of potatoes

300 g of almond milk

unsweetened

250 g of new spinach

200 g of spicy sausage

with pepper and fennel

80 g of spring onions

40 g of almonds in their skin

extra virgin olive oil, salt

Preparation

For the spinach soup recipe, chop the spring onions and fry them in a saucepan with 1 tablespoon of oil; add the peeled potatoes cut into thin slices, 300 g of water and the almond milk; cook for 15 minutes. Add the spinach, salt, cook for another 5 minutes, then blend everything until you obtain a cream. Shell the sausage and toast. Cut the almonds into slices and toast them. Serve the cream with the sausage and almonds. Garnish to taste with baby spinach leaves, a drizzle of oil and freshly ground black pepper.

GNOCCHI WITH STARCH AND VEGETABLE SAUCE

Time 1h 20 min

ingredients

4 people servings

1 kg of red potatoes

200 g of potato starch

Nutmeg

salt

Vegetable Ragu

Preparation

For the gnocchi with starch recipe, wash the potatoes and cook as you prefer, as indicated in the previous recipes; pass them through a potato masher and mix with the starch, a pinch of salt and plenty of grated nutmeg. Form loaves of 2 cm in diameter and cut them into 23 cm pieces; roll under the palm of your hand forming balls. Cook these gnocchi in a large pot of boiling salted water two or three times. Drain them and season them to taste. We prepared a vegetable ragout. Tip: these, like all other doughs, can be flavored to taste with saffron, turmeric, squid ink and tomato paste.

RISOTTO WITH CANDIED CEDAR CAPERS AND SAGE

Time 1h 15min

ingredients

6 servings

480 g of wholemeal Carnaroli rice

100 grams of sugar

80 grams of butter

60 g of parmesan, 1 citron

Rice flour

desalted capers

lemon, sage

White wine vinegar

Preparation

For the recipe for risotto with candied citron, capers and sage, blanch the citron peel for a few moments. Dissolve the sugar with 150 g of water and the juice of 1/2 citron on the heat; add the citrus peel to the syrup and after 1 minute turn off the heat. Let everything cool, then cut the zest into strips. Toast the rice in a fat-free saucepan for a few minutes; wet it with 1 ladle of boiling water and cook it for 4045 minutes, adding a little boiling water little by little. Meanwhile, heat the peanut oil; Flour 30 sage leaves with rice flour and fry them for a few seconds. Drain them and place them on kitchen paper to dry. Salt them lightly when using. Finally, mix the risotto with the butter, parmesan and 1 tablespoon of vinegar and season with salt. Add the grated zest of 1/2 lemon and a drizzle of extra virgin olive oil.

PENNE WITH PUMPKIN AND GORGONZOLA

Time 45 min

ingredients

6 servings

600 g of pumpkin pulp

500 g penne

200g of gorgonzola

60 g of pumpkin seeds

1 pc shallot

extra virgin olive oil

salt

Preparation

For the recipe for penne with pumpkin and gorgonzola, cut the pumpkin pulp into coarse cubes. Finely slice the shallot and brown it in a pan with a drizzle of oil; add 500 g of pumpkin and 300 g of water. Cover with the lid and cook for 1012 minutes over low heat. Blend everything with 1 tablespoon of oil, adding water if necessary, until you obtain a cream. Toast the pumpkin seeds in a hot pan and keep them aside. Fry the remaining pumpkin cubes in the pan with a drizzle of oil; salt. Cook the pasta al dente, drain it and mix it with the pumpkin cream. Serve, completing with the pumpkin cubes, the chunks of gorgonzola and a handful of pumpkin seeds.

GNOCCHI WITH LAMB SAUCE GINGER AND PEANUTS

Time 1h 30min

ingredients

4 people

500 g of potatoes

500 g of lamb meat

300 grams of tomatoes

200 g of 00 flour

200g peanut butter

200 g of onion

100 g of fresh ginger

30 g of tomato puree

1 chili pepper, rosemary, salt

Preparation

For the recipe for gnocchi with lamb, ginger and peanut sauce, boil the whole potatoes, peel them and mash them with a potato masher; Immediately mix the puree obtained with the flour, adding salt to taste. Flour the work surface and shape the gnocchi, first forming a thread of about 1 cm in diameter with the dough, then cutting it into pieces of about 1 cm; Finally, shape the gnocchi on the tines of a fork. Mix the peanut butter with 400 g of water and blend with an immersion blender, mixing the mixture well. Bring to the boil and cook, stirring with a whisk, for about 5 minutes, until it begins to thicken. Cover with a lid, lower the heat and continue cooking for another 25 minutes, stirring occasionally.

Cut the tomatoes into small pieces; peel the ginger and onion and cut them into small pieces too. Blend everything with the chilli pepper, the needles of a sprig of rosemary and 500 g of water. Cut the lamb meat into chunks and cook it in a saucepan with 15 g of salt and the tomato, onion and ginger blend for about 35 minutes, over medium heat and with the saucepan half-covered. Add the peanut sauce and 200 g of water and continue cooking for another 30 minutes, with the pan partially covered; also add the tomato puree, mix and continue cooking for another 20/25 minutes, always with the pan partially covered. Cook the gnocchi in boiling salted water until they float to the surface; drain them with a slotted spoon, season them with the sauce and serve immediately.

LINGUINE ALLA PUTTANESCA

Time 35 min

ingredients

4 servings

400 g of peeled tomatoes

350 g of linguine

80 g of green olives

40 g of desalted capers

2 anchovy fillets in oil

garlic salt

chili

parsley

extra virgin olive oil

Preparation

For the linguine alla puttanesca recipe, fry 1 clove of garlic, a small piece of chilli pepper and the anchovies in plenty of oil until they melt. Remove the garlic and add the tomatoes, crushing them with a spoon; add the pitted olives and cut the capers into small pieces. Cook for 10/15 minutes. In the meantime, boil the linguine in boiling salted water. Drain them al dente and pour them into the pan with the sauce. Complete the pasta with a handful of chopped parsley and serve.

BORLOTTI AND SPINACH STEW WITH TALEGGIO

Time 1h 45 min

ingredients

6 people servings

400 g of rehydrated borlotti beans

250 g of leaf spinach

150 g of taleggio cheese

100 grams of leek

homemade bread

sage, thyme

tomato concentrate

fresh chili pepper

extra virgin olive oil

salt and pepper

Preparation

For the recipe for stewed borlotti beans and spinach with taleggio cheese, pour the beans into a pressure cooker and add water to cover them by two centimetres. Close the lid and turn the heat on to maximum; when the pan whistles, transfer to the smaller burner and continue cooking for another 12 minutes, with the flame at minimum. Cool the pressure cooker under running water, open it, salt and pepper the beans and let them rest for 10 minutes. Peel the leek and cut it into small pieces. Fry it for 10 minutes over low heat in a saucepan with 1/2 sliced chilli pepper, 60 g of oil, 1 tablespoon of tomato paste, 5 sage leaves and a pinch of salt.

Add it to the beans and simmer for 50 minutes, then turn off and let it rest. Heat a pan with a drizzle of oil and brown the spinach leaves, a few at a time, for a couple of minutes, adding salt to taste. Cut three slices of homemade bread into cubes and brown them in a pan with a drizzle of oil, a pinch of salt and a sprig of thyme, until they are golden and crunchy. Cut the taleggio into ½ cm thick slices; remove the crust and break into slices. Transfer the beans into a baking dish, place the sautéed spinach, gathered in tufts, and the taleggio cheese in pieces on top. Cook at 180°C for 3 minutes. Remove from the oven, complete with the crusty bread cubes and serve.

CREAMED RISOTTO WITH HAZELNUT PASTE

Time 25 min

ingredients

4 people

360 g of Carnaroli rice

25 g of hazelnut paste

10 whole toasted hazelnuts

1 white onion

apple cider vinegar

dry white wine

vegetable broth

extra virgin olive oil

Preparation

For the creamed risotto with hazelnut paste recipe, gently brown the sliced onion in a couple of tablespoons of oil until it has lost all the water and has become translucent. Add the rice and toast it briefly, add 1 glass of white wine and continue cooking by adding some hot vegetable broth. Remove from the heat 2 minutes before the scheduled time. Stir the risotto with the hazelnut paste and add a couple of spoons of rice vinegar to calibrate the acidity. Arrange on plates, finish with a drizzle of oil and, if desired, add chervil and sprouts.

HOMEMADE PASTA AND BEANS

Time 1h 30min

ingredients

6 servings

1 Kg fresh borlotti beans

100 g of 00 flour

100 g of re-milled semolina

durum wheat semolina plus a little

30 g of sliced lard, 2 eggs

1 stalk of celery

1 pc Small carrot

1 pc Small onion

Garlic, Rosemary, Laurel

Tomato concentrate

Extra virgin olive oil

salt and pepper

Preparation

Start by shelling the fresh beans and collecting them in a bowl. Cut the celery, carrot and onion into small cubes. Soften the vegetables in a saucepan with 4 tablespoons of oil and 2 bay leaves for 23 minutes. Then add a spoonful of tomato paste. Cook for 12 minutes, then add 2 liters of cold water and the beans. When it boils, add a sprig of rosemary, cover with the lid and cook for about 30 minutes. Towards the end add salt and pepper. Mix the semolina and flour with the eggs until you obtain a smooth dough. Cover it and let it rest in the refrigerator for 1 hour. Roll out the dough into a thin sheet on a floured surface and cut it into squares with a toothed wheel.

Drain half of the cooked beans. Remove the bay leaves and rosemary and blend the soup until creamy. Add the whole beans to the cream and put back on the heat. When it boils, add the pasta and cook for 3 minutes. Very finely chop half a clove of garlic, the leaves of 2 sprigs of rosemary and the lard. Brown the mixture obtained in a hot pan without any other fat until the lard has melted. Add the browned mixture to the pasta and beans and mix well. Turn off the heat and let cool before serving, with freshly ground pepper.

RISOTTO WITH ROSES

Time 30 min

ingredients

Portions for 2 people

160 g of Arborio rice

50 g of fresh cream

50 g of butter

3 edible rose buds

Rosé wine

Grated Parmesan cheese

Rose water

salt and pepper

Preparation

For the rose risotto recipe, cut the petals of 2 rose buds and clean them by removing the white part at the base, which is a little bitter. Soften half in a saucepan with a knob of butter. Add the rice and toast it for 1 minute, then add 1/2 glass of rosé wine. Salt and add a ladle of boiling water, then cook the rice for 15/18 minutes, adding boiling water little at a time. At the end of cooking, add the remaining petals. Mix the risotto with 1 tablespoon of grated Parmesan, the cream and butter and 1 tablespoon of rose water. Serve the risotto, garnishing it with the petals of the third sprout and completing it with a sprinkling of pepper.

TAGLIOLINI WITH SCAMPI WITH LEMON, FENNEL AND ALMONDS

Time 1h 15min

ingredients

6 people servings

1 kg of scampi

400 g of durum wheat semolina

100 g of 00 flour, 2 eggs

1 onion, 1 carrot

1 stalk of celery

1 lemon, butter

fennel, almonds

dry white wine

extra virgin olive oil, salt

Preparation

Clean the scampi: separate the heads and remove the eyes, which are bitter, and cut them in half lengthwise. Shell the tails, and put the pulp aside in the refrigerator. Prepare coarsely chopped celery, carrot and onion. Brown the heads and shells of the scampi tails in a saucepan with a drizzle of oil, crushing them with a ladle, for 1 minute. Add the chopped vegetables and deglaze with 1/2 glass of wine. Then add 1/2 liter of water and cook over low heat for 18/20 minutes. Filter through a sieve and leave the resulting broth to cool. Mix the durum wheat semolina with the flour. Mix them with the whole eggs and about 160 g of broth. Work the mixture until you obtain a homogeneous mixture.

Leave to rest for 30 minutes in the refrigerator, covered. Roll out the dough into thin sheets and cut them, obtaining tagliolini. For the sauce, sauté the scampi tails in a pan with a knob of butter for 2 minutes. If you want to keep them straight, stick them on a toothpick so that the heat of cooking doesn't cause them to curl. Remove them from the pan and, in the meantime, boil the tagliolini in boiling salted water for 2 minutes. Pour the cooking liquid into the scampi pan with 1 ladle of the remaining broth. Drain the tagliolini and sauté them for 1 minute in the pan, then serve them with the scampi tails. Complete them with the grated lemon zest, fennel and sliced almonds.

NOODLES WITH TAMARIND SAUCE (HYDERABADI SALAN)

Time 1h

ingredients

4 people

500 g egg tagliatelle

50 g of roasted peanuts

40 g of tamarind pulp

2 cloves of garlic, 2 tomatoes

2 green chillies

2 large aubergines

1 onion, 1 lemon

fresh ginger, fresh coriander

cumin seeds, sesame seeds

black mustard seeds

peanut oil, granulated sugar

extra virgin olive oil, salt

Preparation

For the recipe of noodles with tamarind sauce (hyderabadi salan), blanch the tomatoes, remove the peel, cut them into small pieces, also remove the seeds, then chop them. Chop the onion and peppers. Dilute the tamarind pulp in 30 g of water. Blend the onion with the peeled garlic cloves, 35 g of peanuts, the chopped tomatoes, ½ cm of ginger root, the chopped chillies, 2 tablespoons of sesame seeds, ½ teaspoon of cumin seeds, the lemon juice , ½ tablespoon of sugar and the diluted tamarind, until you obtain a smooth paste (if you don't want a too spicy taste, reduce the quantity or eliminate the chillies altogether). Heat 2 tablespoons of extra virgin olive oil in a pan and add ½ teaspoon of black mustard seeds and toast them until the spices begin to crackle; add the blended mixture and leave to flavor over low heat for 1 minute, then add a couple of ladles of water and continue cooking for 15 minutes, stirring occasionally and adding salt. Cut the aubergines into cubes and fry them in plenty of peanut oil for 45 minutes, until golden. Drain them on kitchen paper. Cook the tagliatelle in abundant boiling salted water according to the times indicated on the package; drain them and add them to the sauce with a little of their cooking water. Mix well, leave to flavor for 12 minutes, then add the fried aubergines. Chop the remaining peanuts and distribute over the tagliatelle; complete with a little chopped coriander and a drizzle of extra virgin olive oil.

CITRUS RISOTTO

Time 40 min

ingredients

Portions for 4 people

250 grams of rice

2 mandarins

1 grapefruit

1 shallot

vegetable broth

Grated Parmesan cheese

extra virgin olive oil

butter, salt

Preparation

For the citrus fruit risotto recipe, recover the peels of the citrus fruits, cut them into fillets and blanch them for 2 minutes in boiling water; drain them and let them dry. Cut the segments of 1 mandarin and, if desired, free them from the peel. Chop the shallot and sauté it gently in a large pan with a thin layer of oil. Add the rice, toast it for 1 minute, then blend with the grapefruit juice and 1 mixed mandarin. Cook it for about 15 minutes, gradually adding the vegetable broth. Finally, stir in 60 g of butter and 80 g of grated parmesan. Serve immediately, completing with a little zest and mandarin segments.

PENNE, BROCCOLI HAZELNUTS AND PAPRIKA

Duration 30 min

ingredients

Portions for 4 people

320 g of penne rigate

50 g of toasted peeled hazelnuts

1 broccoli

smoked paprika

extra virgin olive oil, sale

Preparation

For the penne, broccoli, hazelnuts and paprika recipe, prepare the broccoli: separate the florets from the stem. Collect all parts of the stem and twigs, and partially peel them, removing only the most fibrous external factors. Boil the florets and the rest beautiful leaves for 34 minutes (they will be used to complete the dishes); drain them with a slotted spoon (the florets are slightly al dente). Cut the stems and larger florets into chunks and cook them in the same water until tender. Drain them with a slotted spoon and blend with 30 g of hazelnuts and a couple of spoons of oil, salt and the tip of a teaspoon of smoked paprika; adjust the consistency, which must be creamy: if necessary, add a little cooking water. Heat the cream in a large pan. Drain the broccoli in the cooking water, boil the penne, drain them al dente and toss them in the broccoli cream. Arrange them on plates and complete them with the florets, the leaves blanched for a few moments in boiling water, the remaining coarsely chopped hazelnuts and the smoked paprika.

HOME RICE (ARROZ CASERO) WITH TOMATO AND CHILI PEPPER

Time 35 min

ingredients

Servings for 6 people

800 g of ripe tomatoes

400 g of Carnaroli rice

6 basil leaves

2 stalks of celery

1 onion

1 spring onion

dried chili pepper

salt extra virgin olive oil

Preparation

For the recipe for homemade rice (Arroz Casero) with tomato and chilli pepper, prepare the broth by bringing 500/600 g of water to the boil with the peeled onion, celery stalks and a pinch of salt: simmer for 15/20 minutes to let them flavor. Blend the raw tomatoes with the spring onion, eliminating the root and the green part. Rinse the rice to remove the starch, then dry it with kitchen paper and toast it in a large non-stick pan (ø 25/30 cm) with 45 tablespoons of oil for 23 minutes on high heat. Add the tomato and spring onion sauce to the rice, a pinch of salt, a pinch of chilli (depending on your taste), 23 basil leaves and cook over a low heat for 15 minutes, spread the rice well in the pan with the back of the spoon and never cover it; once the sauce has dried, add a little broth at a time (a ladle) and continue for another 8/10 minutes: it must remain slightly al dente, like the rice in paella. Bring the rice to the table, completing it with more basil leaves and, if you like, more chilli pepper. The ingredient: as chilli we used chile de árbol, a medium spicy Mexican variety. It can be replaced with other types as long as it is in flakes, which are tastier, and not in powder form.

FILEJA TROPEA (CALABRIAN)

Time 1h

ingredients

8 people

600 g of 00 flour

400 g of durum wheat flour

Fresh tomato sauce

extra virgin olive oil

basil

salt

Preparation

For the Calabrian fileja di Tropea recipe, mix the two flours and sift them on the work surface. Form a crater in the center and start pouring 500 g of room temperature water little by little. Knead first with the tines of a fork, then with your hands. Work vigorously with the palms of your hands for about 20 minutes, until you obtain a smooth and elastic dough. Take some pieces and shape them into cords of about 5 cm; then slide them along a metal wire (fileja) until you obtain an 8/10 cm macaroni. Gradually arrange the fileja on a floured surface; cook in salted water for 60 minutes. Season them with tomato sauce and basil leaves.

LINGUINE WITH FISH SAUCE

Time 1h 30 min

ingredients

Servings for 6 people

480 g of linguine

500 g of tomato puree

250 g 1 small octopus already cleaned

150 g of already cleaned cuttlefish

150 g of peeled prawn tails

150 g of gurnard fillets

100 g white fish pulp

3 shallots chopped

1 cleaned squid, 120 g of celery

carrot, onion, 100 g of dry white wine

1 clove of garlic, 1 fresh chilli pepper

extra virgin olive oil

chopped parsley

fish soup

Preparation

For the linguine with fish sauce recipe, cut the fish, crustaceans and molluscs into chunks. Brown the celery, carrot and onion in a saucepan with oil and garlic, then add all the fish, deglaze with the wine, let it evaporate, add the tomato puree, 1 ladle of fish broth and the chilli pepper cut in half in the direction of length; lower the heat and cook for about 40 minutes; Finally, remove the chilli and garlic. Cook the linguine in boiling salted water, drain them al dente and season them in the saucepan with the ragù, adding 1 ladle of cooking water and the chopped parsley.

PEN, CUTTLEFISH AND BOTTARGA

Time 50 min + 1h marination

ingredients

4 people

400 g of cleaned cuttlefish

300 grams of tomatoes

320 g of half penne

40 grams of fennel

40 g of bottarga

1 spicy green chili pepper

dry white wine

thyme, parsley

extra virgin olive oil

salt and pepper

Preparation

For the penne, cuttlefish and bottarga recipe, cut the cherry tomatoes into small pieces and season them with 35/40 g of oil, freshly ground pepper and chopped green pepper. Leave to marinate for 1 hour. Place the cuttlefish in a pan, cover them with cold water, and flavor with a splash of white wine, 23 sprigs of thyme and a sprig of parsley. Bring to a boil and cook for 67 minutes; let the cuttlefish cool in their water in a covered pan, then cut them into thin strips. Bring a pan of water to the boil, season it with the chopped fennel and cook the pasta, drain it al dente. Let it cool by spreading it on a tray with the cooking fennel and season everything with a drizzle of oil. Transfer the half penne with the fennel into a salad bowl; add the cuttlefish strips, the marinated tomato, the flaked bottarga and season with salt.

LINGUINE WITH RAW PRAWN

Time 25 min

ingredients

4 people

350 g of prawn tails

Linguine 320 g

2 fresh chillies

4 whole prawns

garlic

chopped pistachios

extra virgin olive oil

salt

Preparation

For the raw scampi linguine recipe, shell the scampi tails and wash them, open them in half lengthwise and place them on a sheet of cling film. Cover them with another sheet of cling film and mash them with a meat tenderizer, obtaining a sort of carpaccio. Shell the whole prawns, remove the heads and keep the tails. Boil the linguine in boiling salted water. In a pan, heat 4 tablespoons of oil with 1 chopped clove of garlic and the chillies, deseeded and cut into small pieces. Cook for 2 minutes, then add 2 tablespoons of chopped pistachios. Drain the pasta and sauté it in this oil. Serve it with the prawn carpaccio and garnish with the tails kept whole.

PIZZOCCHERI

Time 1h 30min

ingredients

Portions for 4 people

The Pizzoccheri

400 g of buckwheat flour

100 g of 00 flour

salt

the Seasoning

250 grams of potatoes

200 g of cabbage leaves

120 grams of butter

180 g of Asiago cheese

100 g Grana Padano

2 cloves of garlic, salt

Preparation

For the pizzoccheri, mix the buckwheat flour and the 00 flour with about 250 g of water and a pinch of salt until you obtain a firm and smooth dough. Leave to rest covered for 30 minutes. Then roll it out into a 23 mm thick sheet and cut out the pizzoccheri: strips approximately 5 mm wide and 78 cm long. For the dressing Cut the asiago into thin slices. Peel the potatoes and cut them into chunks. Clean the cabbage, remove the central rib and cut the leaves into small pieces. Boil the potatoes in chunks in a large pan of boiling salted water for about 5 minutes, add the cabbage cut into strips and the pizzoccheri and cook for about ten minutes.

Meanwhile, heat the butter in a small saucepan with the garlic cloves until it starts to colour. Drain the pizzoccheri, cabbage and potatoes with a slotted spoon and arrange the first layer in a baking dish; sprinkle them with the sliced cheeses and grated parmesan, then drain the other pizzoccheri and proceed in layers until the ingredients are used up. Pour the golden butter over the pizzoccheri and serve immediately.

SICILIAN CANNELLONI

Time 1h

ingredients

Portions for 4 people

800 g of beef stew

500 g pasta sheets

with egg for fresh lasagna

200 g grated parmesan

2 eggs

extra virgin olive oil

salt

Pepper

Preparation

For the Sicilian cannoli recipe, cut the pasta into rectangles of approximately 8 x 12 cm. Dip them for a few moments in boiling salted water, drain them and spread them out, without overlapping them, on some tea towels; let them cool. Chop the stew rather finely with a knife, flavor it with 100 g of grated parmesan, mix and season with salt and pepper. Distribute the meat on the pasta rectangles and wrap starting from the short side to obtain the cannelloni. Place them in a baking dish greased with oil, sprinkle with the rest of the grated parmesan and cook in the oven at 180°C for 15/20 minutes. Remove from the oven and sprinkle with the beaten eggs, bake again under the grill for 78 minutes, remove from the oven and serve.

SHELLS APRICOT AND PAPRIKA ON CHICKPEA CREAM

Time 40 min

ingredients

4 people

350 g of shell pasta

220 g of drained boiled chickpeas

120 g of drained boiled black chickpeas

6 apricots

Spicy paprika

basil, lemon

extra virgin olive oil

salt, pepper, ice

Preparation

For the shells recipe, add the apricots and paprika to the chickpea cream, and cook the shells in boiling salted water. Drain them, season them with a drizzle of oil and let them cool, spreading them out on a tray. Blend the chickpeas with 80 g of their preserving liquid and 50 g of water, the juice of 1/2 lemon, salt, pepper and 2 tablespoons of oil, obtaining a cream. Brown the black chickpeas in a pan with 2 tablespoons of oil and a pinch of paprika powder. Blend a sprig of basil leaves with 1 ice cube and 40 g of oil. Collect the pasta in a bowl and season it with the black chickpeas and their oil, add the chopped apricots, then place everything on the chickpea cream. Finish with a little paprika.

BAKED ZITI

Time 1h 15min

ingredients

Servings for 6 people

500 g of ziti

500 g of tomato puree

400 g of minced beef pulp

250 g of grated scamorza

2 hard boiled eggs

1 onion

Grated Parmesan cheese

extra virgin olive oil

salt and pepper

Preparation

For the baked ziti recipe, chop the onion, fry it in a pan with a thin layer of oil, season with 200 g of beef pulp, then add the tomato puree and salt. Cook the sauce for 35 minutes. Mix the remaining pulp with 30 g of parmesan, 2 tablespoons of oil, salt and pepper. Form balls the size of an olive. Sauté the meatballs in the pan with a thin layer of oil, allowing them to brown evenly, then cook in the sauce for 5 minutes, keeping some aside. Boil the ziti al dente; drain them, toss them in the sauce and transfer them to a baking dish. Mix with the scamorza and the slices of hard-boiled egg; distribute the meatballs kept aside on the surface, sprinkle with parmesan and bake at 190°C for 20 minutes. Also good warm or at room temperature.

RISOTTO WITH I
GREEN PEPPERS

Time 30 min

ingredients

Portions for 4 people

320 g of Vialone Nano rice

80 grams of butter

80 g Pecorino

60 g of rocket

2 green peppers

dry white wine

Peanut oil

salt

Preparation

For the green pepper risotto recipe, dry toast the rice with a pinch of salt. Deglaze it with a splash of white wine and cook it for about 16 minutes, adding boiling water, little at a time. Clean the peppers, removing seeds and white filaments. Keep one aside for decoration and blend the others in a centrifuge with the rocket. Fry the pepper kept aside in hot peanut oil for 2 minutes, drain it, remove the skin and cut it into small pieces. Stir the risotto with the pepper juice (keep some), the butter and the pecorino. Complete with drops of centrifuged juice, fried chilli pepper and rocket to taste.

RISOTTO WITH FONTINA AND APPLES

Time 25 min

ingredients

Portions for 4 people

350 g of Carnaroli rice

150 g Fontina DOP

130 grams of butter

50 g grated parmesan

3 green apples

vegetable broth

kirsch, salt

Pepper

Preparation

For the Fontina and apple risotto recipe, toast the rice with 50 g of butter and a pinch of salt for 2/3 minutes. Pour in the kirsch and add 1 ladle of broth. Cook, adding a little broth at a time (about 1 liter), for 15 minutes. Stir the risotto with the remaining butter, the grated parmesan and the diced fontina. Also add 2 peeled and diced apples. Cover the rice and let it rest for 3/4 minutes. Cut the remaining apple into thin slices. Season with salt and pepper and serve, completing with the apple slices and, if desired, with the fried sage.

RISOTTO WITH BLUEBERRIES, BLACKBERRIES AND FONTINA

Time 35 min

ingredients

4 people

320 grams of rice

250 g of blueberries

200 g of butter

180 g of fontina

125 g of blackberries

2 shallots, salt

White wine vinegar

dry white wine

extra virgin olive oil

Preparation

For the blueberry, blackberry and fontina risotto recipe, peel and chop the shallot. Heat 5 tablespoons of vinegar in a saucepan with ½ glass of white wine and salt. When it comes to the boil, add the shallot, after 24 minutes add the cold butter, remove from the heat and whisk. Cut the blueberries in half and place them in a small pan with 4 tablespoons of very hot oil and 2 pinches of salt; mash them a little and brown them for 23 minutes over high heat. Dry toast the rice with a pinch of salt; when it is hot add the whipped butter; after 1 minute pour in hot unsalted water, after another 2 minutes add the blueberry sauce and cook, adding the necessary hot water (it will take 16 minutes in total). At the end of cooking, stir in 60 g of fontina;

ITALIAN PAELLA

Time 30 min

ingredients

6 people

500 g of cleaned mussels

400 g of cleaned squid

400 g of peeled prawn tails

400 g of Arborio rice

2 sachets of saffron

1 onion

fish soup

extra virgin olive oil

parsley, lemon

Preparation

For the Italian paella recipe, chop the onion and brown it in a saucepan with a drizzle of oil. Toast the rice for 2 minutes, add 800 g of broth and the saffron. Bring to the boil, cover with the lid, reduce the heat to minimum and cook for 10/12 minutes. Cut the squid into rings, the tufts in half. Add them to the rice together with the prawn tails (keep the best ones aside) and cook for another 3/4 minutes. Open the mussels in the pan with a drizzle of oil. Serve the rice on a tray, complete with the prawn tails, mussels, chopped parsley and lemon wedges.

RECIPES
SECOND DISHES

RABBIT BREADED WITH DROPS OF BALSAMIC

Time 30 min + 12h

resting time for the marinade

ingredients

4 people

500 g rabbit meat

2 eggs, sage

rosemary, lemon

dry white wine

flour, breadcrumbs

Peanut oil

balsamic vinegar

salt and pepper

Preparation

For the recipe for breaded rabbit with drops of balsamic vinegar, cut the rabbit into bite-sized pieces and place them in a bowl with a sprig of sage, a few sprigs of rosemary, 34 slices of lemon, 250 g of white wine, pepper. Cover and leave to marinate for 12 hours in a cool place. Drain the morsels from the marinade, dry them with kitchen paper, then flour them and dip them in the beaten eggs with a pinch of salt and dip them in the breadcrumbs. Fry them in plenty of peanut oil, at 165°C, for about 2 minutes. Drain them on kitchen paper, drain them and serve them immediately, completing with drops of balsamic vinegar.

GRATIN COD

Time 50 min

ingredients

4 servings

800 g of desalted cod fillet

200 g of stale breadcrumbs

40 g of walnut kernels

40 g of raisins

8 dried figs

parsley

garlic

extra virgin olive oil

Preparation

For the gratin cod recipe, clean the cod, remove all the bones and place it in a baking dish suitable for going from the oven to the table. Coarsely blend the breadcrumbs. Chop the figs, nuts and raisins. Finely chop a sprig of parsley with 1 clove of garlic and distribute part of it over the cod. Mix the remaining mixture with the breadcrumbs and the chopped dried fruit. Season the fish with a drizzle of cooked must, then cover it with the bread and dried fruit mixture. Season with a drizzle of oil and bake at 180°C for about 20 minutes.

BORLOTTI MEATLOAF, GREEN BEANS AND CHEESE, WRAPPED IN HAM

Time 1h 45min

ingredients

68 people

350 g of boiled borlotti beans

300 grams of potatoes

120 g of robiola type cheese

100 g of green beans

100 g of sliced raw ham

30 g of parmesan

1 egg, marjoram

extra virgin olive oil

salt and pepper

Preparation

For the meatloaf recipe with borlotti beans, green beans and cheese wrapped in ham, boil the potatoes in boiling water for about 40 minutes. Clean the green beans and boil them in boiling salted water for 5 minutes, then drain them. Blend the beans with 3 tablespoons of oil using an immersion blender. Mash the potatoes and add them to the bean cream, together with the egg, grated parmesan, salt, pepper, a sprig of chopped marjoram and chopped green beans. Mix everything until the ingredients are combined. Lay the ham slices next to each other on a sheet of baking paper, slightly overlapping each other.

You will obtain a rectangle: turn it so that the ham slices are vertical in front of you; arrange the meatloaf mixture on the base. Create a groove in the center and fill it with the cheese, then close the mixture giving it a cylindrical shape. Finally, roll it in the slices of ham, using the baking paper. Wrap the meatloaf in paper, as if it were a candy. Grease the outside with a drizzle of oil, place it in a baking dish and bake at 180°C for 35 minutes; then open the paper and cook for another 78 minutes.

ROAST CAPITONE

Time 1h + 1h marination

ingredients

Portions for 4 people

1 kg of capitone fish slices

200 g of breadcrumbs

200 g of cleaned broccoli

200 g of cleaned Romanesco broccoli

120 g of carrots

100 g of cleaned black cabbage

80 g of white vinegar

3 lemons, 2 red onions

1 beetroot

thyme, marjoram

rosemary, bay leaf

extra virgin olive oil

salt and pepper

Preparation

For the roasted capitone recipe, place the capitone slices in a bowl and add the juice of 2 lemons, the vinegar, 100 g of oil, two pinches of salt, pepper and 4-5 chopped bay leaves. Mix everything well and leave to marinate covered for about 1 hour. Blend the breadcrumbs with the leaves of a sprig of thyme, one of marjoram and the needles of a sprig of rosemary. Dip the pieces of capitone in the flavored bread and thread them onto the skewers, alternating the pieces of capitone with half slices of lemon.

Assemble 4 skewers and place them on a baking tray covered with baking paper. Bake them at 180°C for about 40 minutes. In the meantime, prepare the vegetables: peel the turnip, cut it into 4 segments and boil them in boiling water for about 35 minutes. Peel the carrots and cut them lengthwise; cut the broccoli into tufts. Dip them in boiling salted water, after 1 minute add the black cabbage, and after 3 minutes drain everything in cold water. Peel the onion, cut it into petals, then boil them for 5 minutes in the water in which you cooked the beets. Remove the skewers from the oven and serve them with the vegetables, seasoned to taste with a drizzle of oil and a few pinches of salt.

CHICKEN AND PORCINI ROLLERS GINGER IN KATAIFI PASTE

Time 40 min

ingredients

8 people

400 g 8 slices of chicken breast

180 g of porcini mushrooms

150 g of mayonnaise

125 g of Greek yogurt

90 g of bread for sandwiches

fresh ginger

kataifi dough

chives, basil

Peanut oil

extra virgin olive oil, salt

Preparation

For the recipe for chicken, porcini and porcini mushroom rolls with ginger, in kataifi paste, remove the crust from the bread and blend it. Clean the mushrooms and cut them into small pieces. Brown in a pan with a drizzle of extra virgin olive oil, 34 slices of ginger and a pinch of salt for 23 minutes. Turn it off and let it cool. Finely chop the mushrooms, finely chop the browned ginger and add everything to the bread. Season with salt and add 1 tablespoon of sliced chives to this filling.

Lightly beat the chicken breast slices to thin them, fill them in the center with a knob of filling and close like a roll. Wrap each chicken roll in kataifi dough; fry them for 3 minutes in peanut oil at 170°C, with 2/3 slices of ginger. Drain them on kitchen paper. Mix the mayonnaise with the Greek yogurt, a small piece of grated ginger and a few chopped basil leaves. Serve the rolls with the ginger mayonnaise.

RABBIT WITH NUTMEG
AND BAKED PUMPKIN

Time 55 min

ingredients

4 people

2 rabbit saddles

600 g 4 slices of yellow pumpkin

200 g Berrettina pumpkin pulp

Nutmeg

wild watercress

extra virgin olive oil

salt

Preparation

For the rabbit with nutmeg and baked pumpkin recipe, deboned (or have the butcher do it for) the rabbit saddles, obtaining 4 defatted loins. Also, keep your kidneys. Arrange the pumpkin slices and chopped pulp on a baking tray, season everything with a drizzle of oil and salt and cook in the oven at 160°C for about 15 minutes. Remove from the oven and set the slices aside. Mash the pulp with a potato masher, then work it with a drizzle of oil until you obtain a cream. Keep him warm. Brown the rabbit loins in a hot pan with a drizzle of oil, so that they brown on all sides.

Sprinkle with plenty of grated nutmeg, place them on a baking tray and bake at 160°C for 67 minutes. Remove the rabbit from the oven and let it rest in the heat for at least 15 minutes. Keep the cooking sauce aside and mix it with a drizzle of oil. Separate the ribs from the pulp, cut the latter into chunks and the kidneys in half. Serve the rabbit and kidneys together with the pumpkin slices and cream and complete with the wild watercress leaves and the cooking sauce.

SCALLOPS WITH GRAPES AND MUSHROOMS

Time 20 min

ingredients

4 people

300 g of fresh porcini mushrooms

120 g of seedless white grapes

120 g of seedless red grapes

12 scallops

Butter

garlic

parsley

salt and pepper

Preparation

For the scallops with grapes and mushrooms recipe, roast the scallops in a pan, in a knob of foaming butter, over high heat, turning them on both sides, for 23 minutes. Salt them lightly. Transfer the shellfish to a plate and keep the cooking juices. Clean the baking tray with kitchen paper. Clean the mushrooms and cut them into small pieces. Cut the larger grapes in half. Add a new knob of butter to the pan and sauté the porcini mushrooms and grapes with 1 crushed garlic clove and a pinch of salt for 3 minutes. Put the scallops and their cooking juices back in the pan, mix, remove the garlic and pepper and serve with chopped parsley.

LUCIANA-STYLE FISHERMAN AND CRISPY ARTICHOKES

Time 1h 10min

ingredients

Servings for 46 people

1kg monkfish slice

150 g of tomato puree

80 g of green olives

30 g of desalted capers

3 artichokes, 1 lemon

1 clove of garlic

Marjoram

thyme, celery

extra virgin olive oil

peanut oil, salt

Preparation

For the Luciana monkfish recipe, clean the monkfish slice and remove the cuticles; turn it over, make two incisions along the central bone, remove it and keep it aside. Tie the monkfish steak like a roast: in this way it will maintain greater succulence during cooking. Prepare an aromatic bunch with a sprig of marjoram, a sprig of thyme and a stalk of celery. Heat a pan, preferably cast iron or steel, with 2 tablespoons of oil; brown the roasted monkfish for 1 minute, add salt, add the peeled and crushed garlic and the aromatic bunch, the olives,

Add the desalted capers, then cover everything with the tomato puree; add 50 g of water, the monkfish bone, cover and cook for 50 minutes over low heat. Clean the artichokes, eliminating the thorns and the internal beard; cut them into wedges and gradually immerse them in water acidulated with lemon juice. Fry the artichokes in plenty of peanut oil for 56 minutes, then drain them on kitchen paper and sabatelli. Slice the roasted monkfish and serve it with its sauce and crunchy artichokes.

**DUCK BREAST E
PORCINI SIDE SIDE**

Time 40 min

ingredients

4 servings

1 duck breast

350 g of porcini mushrooms

200 g of Renetta apple

1 pc shallot

Rosemary

parsley

garlic

White wine

vegetable broth, lemon

extra virgin olive oil

butter, salt, pepper

Preparation

For the duck breast and porcini side dish recipe, clean the porcini mushrooms, separating the stems and caps. Finely chop the shallot; cut the apple into cubes, and the stems of the porcini mushrooms into slices, and brown everything in a pan with a drizzle of oil. Score the duck skin like a grill to prevent it from curling during cooking. Lightly pepper the breast and brown it in an oven-safe pan with a drizzle of hot oil and a sprig of rosemary, for 1 and a half minutes on the skin side, then turn it over, add 1/2 glass of white wine, add half of the whole porcini mushroom caps and bake at 200°C for 78 minutes or a little more, depending on the degree of cooking you prefer. Remove the breast from the oven and let it rest for 10 minutes wrapped in aluminum foil. Blend the cooking juices with 40 g of vegetable broth and the remaining chapels to obtain a sauce. Cut a couple of cloves of garlic and mince them with a sprig of parsley. In the pan where you cooked the meat, melt a knob of butter with a little grated lemon zest and the chopped mixture, add the white wine and when it has almost evaporated, add the sauce, salt and pepper. Serve the sliced duck breast with the apple and porcini stalks, the caps and the sauce.

CHICKEN IN CREAM AND PORCINI

Time 45 min

ingredients

4 people

1.5kg 1 chicken

500 g of fresh cream

400 g of fresh porcini mushrooms

grappa 150 g

1 onion, garlic and butter

rosemary, sage

parsley

extra virgin olive oil

salt and pepper

Preparation

For the chicken with cream and porcini recipe, cut the chicken into 8 pieces and brown it over high heat in a pan with 1 clove of garlic, without adding fat. Scented with some sage and rosemary leaves. Once cooked, after 45 minutes, pour in the brandy, salt and pepper. Cover with the lid and leave to cook for about 20 minutes. Chop the onion and sauté it in a large pan with a knob of butter, a drizzle of oil and a pinch of salt. Add the cream, bring it to the boil, turn off the heat and season with salt and pepper. Clean the mushrooms and cut them into small pieces.

Brown them in a pan with a drizzle of oil and 1 clove of garlic with the peel, for 23 minutes. Season with salt and pepper, then add a small, finely chopped clove of garlic. Chop half of the browned porcini mushrooms and add them to the cream. Also add the chicken, together with part of its cooking juices, and cook everything for 5 minutes over low heat, with the lid on. Finally add the remaining mushrooms and serve with fresh parsley.

STUFFED COURGETTES

Time 1h 40min

ingredients

6 people

1 kg 6 courgettes

500 g of diced veal meat

50 g of raw ham

40 g of dry breadcrumbs

20 g grated parmesan

1 egg

1 stalk of celery

1 carrot

1/2 onion, milk

parsley

dry white wine

extra virgin olive oil

salt and pepper

Preparation

For the stuffed courgettes recipe, cut the courgettes horizontally, obtaining a thicker part, the base, and a thinner part, the lid. Generously empty the thickest part and keep the pulp obtained. Blanch the bases and lids in boiling salted water for 2 minutes; Drain them on kitchen paper. Chop the celery, carrot and onion and sauté them in a large pan with 3 tablespoons of oil for 2/3 minutes. Add the veal pulp and brown it over a high heat, being careful not to burn the vegetables; after 5/7 minutes add 1/2 glass of white wine and 1 ladle of water; lower the heat, cover and cook for about 20 minutes, then add the courgette pulp, another ladle of water, salt, pepper and cook for another 15 minutes. Finally, drain the meat (keep the cooking juices), chop and mix it with the egg, parmesan, chopped ham, breadcrumbs soaked in milk and squeezed out, 1 tablespoon of chopped parsley, salt and pepper. Stuff the bases of the courgettes with the mixture, close them with the lids and secure them with a few turns of kitchen string. Place the courgettes in a baking dish, and add the cooking juices and a drop of water, if necessary. Bake at 180°C for 20/25 minutes.

PUMPKIN CHICKPEAS, AND MUSHROOM MEATLOAF

Time 1.30 minutes

ingredients

4 people

1.5 kg Delica pumpkin

300 g of porcini mushrooms

230 g of boiled chickpeas

150 grams of spinach

2 eggs, thyme

garlic, parsley

Grated Parmesan cheese

breadcrumbs, vinegar

extra virgin olive oil

salt and pepper

Preparation

Cut the pumpkin into small pieces, remove the seeds, place them on a baking tray covered with baking paper, season with oil, sprigs of thyme, salt and pepper and place in the oven at 180°C for 1 hour. Remove from the oven and recover the pulp; cut it into pieces and blend with chickpeas, eggs, salt, pepper and 1 tablespoon of vinegar. Blanch the spinach in boiling salted water, drain and spread out on sheets of kitchen paper to dry. Clean the mushrooms and cut them into chunks; Brown in a pan with a drizzle of oil, 1 clove of garlic, salt and pepper for 3 minutes, then complete with a sprig of chopped parsley.

Spread the pumpkin mixture on a sheet of baking paper brushed with oil, using another sheet and a rolling pin, creating a rectangular base. Trim the edges and cover the rectangle of pasta with spinach. Then distribute the mushrooms on the shortest side of the rectangle and from there roll up the meatloaf using the baking paper. Mix 1 tablespoon of breadcrumbs with 1 tablespoon of grated parmesan and sprinkle the surface of the meatloaf, then bake at 170°C for about 25 minutes.

STUFFED CHICKEN TIGHS WITH EXOTIC COCONUT MILK SAUCE

Time 1h 40min

ingredients

4 servings

For the chicken

4 chicken thighs

180 g of boiled chestnuts

160 g salami paste

Rosemary, thyme, salt

extra virgin olive oil, pepper

For the curry

400 g of coconut milk, 10 g of parsley

5 g of fresh ginger, 1 pc of green chilli

1 lime, fresh coriander

dried coriander, cumin, salt

extra virgin olive oil

Preparation

Deboning the thighs: with a sharp knife, cut the flesh all around the bone until it is completely free. Turn the pulp inside out like a glove, grab the bone, cut through the rest of the connective tissue, and then peel it away from the thigh. Only one piece will remain, on the outside. Coarsely chop the chestnuts with the leaves of a sprig of rosemary and two sprigs of thyme. Mix everything with the salami paste and 1 tablespoon of oil until you obtain a compact mixture. Season the inside of the chicken thighs with salt and pepper, stuff them with the filling;

put them together and tie them tightly with a few turns of kitchen twine. Place the legs on a baking tray lined with baking paper; season them with salt, pepper and a drizzle of oil. Cook them in a static oven at 190°C for about 50 minutes. For curries, divide the chilli pepper in half and remove the stem and seeds; coarsely chopped with parsley and ginger. Blend everything with 20 g of coconut milk, the grated zest of 1/2 lime, the juice of 1 lime, 1 teaspoon of dried coriander, 1/2 teaspoon of cumin, 23 sprigs of fresh coriander and a drizzle of oil . Simmer the remaining coconut milk for 23 minutes. Let it cool and then mix with the smoothie; salt, if necessary. Serve the chicken legs with the curry, decorating as desired.

MULLETS WITH HAM

Time 45 min

+ 1h of marinade

ingredients

4 people

8 red mullets

5 slices of raw ham

sage (20 leaves)

butter, lemon

bread crumbs

extra virgin olive oil

salt and pepper

Preparation

For the recipe for red mullets with ham, carefully clean the red mullets: gut them under a jet of running water, then pass them through knife along the bone, help yourself with a finger and separate the bone from the pulp on the other side too; break the bone on the head side and cut the hairline on the tail side with scissors; finally rinse the red mullets and place them in a baking dish. Prepare a marinade with the juice of 1/42 lemon, 4 tablespoons of oil, salt and pepper and pour over the red mullets in the baking dish; cover with cling film and place in the fridge to flavor for 1 hour. Sprinkle 8/10 sage leaves and the bottom of another baking dish with butter. Stuff the belly of the mullet with a buttered sage leaf; roll the fish in breadcrumbs. Divide the ham slices in half. Arrange the red mullet alternating with the ham in the pan, sprinkle with the marinade and add the remaining sage leaves. Bake at 180°C for 15/20 minutes.

SEAFOOD SALAD

Time 30 minutes

ingredients

4 people

12 peeled red prawns

12 scampi

12 medium calamari cut into pieces

4 medium potatoes, diced

1 shallot sliced

candied lemon

parsley

vegetable broth

extra virgin olive oil

salt and pepper

Preparation

For the seafood salad recipe, brown the shallot in a little oil, then add the potatoes, cover with the hot vegetable broth and cook until cooked: blend and season with salt and pepper. Shell prawns and scampi without removing the head; steam them for a maximum of 45 minutes and do the same with the calamari. Distribute the potato cream on the plates and complete with scampi, prawns and calamari. Season with a drizzle of oil and decorate with aromatic herbs, candied lemon wedges, puffed fregola and potato chips.

VEGETABLE SKEWERS WITH OKRA

Time 45 min

ingredients

4 people

500g fresh okra

200g chilli sticks

200 g carrot sticks

100 g of breadcrumbs

30 g of shelled walnuts

4 medium cabbage leaves

1 golden apple

curry, salt

smoked sweet paprika

extra virgin olive oil

Preparation

For the okra vegetable skewers recipe, blanch the okra in boiling salted water for 45 minutes after it has started to boil again, then drain it in cold water, drain it and dry it gently with a cloth. Blanch the other vegetables too. Blend the breadcrumbs with 1 tablespoon of curry, 1 teaspoon of paprika, the walnuts, a couple of tablespoons of oil and salt; you will have to obtain a fairly fine mixture. Assemble 4 skewers alternating the okra, apple segments and vegetable sticks on each stick (in season you can add 200 g of white asparagus); Grease them with oil and pass them in the bread mixture. Brown the skewers in a pan on both sides until golden brown. Sprinkle it with salt just before enjoying it.

BREADED EGG, BEANS AND CRISPY PLATANA

Time 45 minutes

ingredients

4 people

300 g of tomato puree

250 g 1 ripe plantain

150g canned borlotti beans

75 g of breadcrumbs

75 g corn snack smoothie

70 g of butter, salt

30 g of tomato puree

6 fresh organic eggs

Peanut oil

extra virgin olive oil

Preparation

For the breaded egg, beans and crispy plantain recipe, place the boiled beans in a saucepan for about 10/15 minutes and season with salt. Add the tomato paste and cook for another 5 minutes. Cook the tomato puree with the butter and a drizzle of extra virgin olive oil for 10 minutes, then blend everything with an immersion blender. Season the beans with this sauce. Peel the plantain, cut it into oblique slices, immerse them in salted water and leave to rest for 10 minutes, then drain and dry them on kitchen paper.

Fry them in plenty of hot peanut oil for about 5 minutes, until they are golden and crispy. Cook 4 eggs in boiling water for 5 minutes. Shell and coat them in breadcrumbs, dipping in 2 beaten eggs, then in breadcrumbs, then again in beaten eggs, and finally in corn powder. Fry the eggs in plenty of hot peanut oil, one at a time, for 1 minute, turning them to brown them evenly. Drain them on kitchen paper. Serve them with beans and bananas.

SQUID STUFFED WITH RICOTTA AND CATALONIA

Time 50 min

ingredients

4 servings

8 pcs. squid

500 g of ricotta

Catalonia 300 g

30 g of breadcrumbs

4 anchovy fillets in oil

garlic, marjoram

extra virgin olive oil

salt and pepper

Preparation

For the recipe for squid stuffed with ricotta and catalonia, wash the catalonia and remove it the hardest part of the stem and cut it into small pieces. Melt the anchovies in a pan with a drizzle of oil and 1 clove of garlic. Add the catalonia and cook for about 3 minutes. Clean the squid, separating the sacs from the head with the tentacles. Remove the beak and eyes; remove the internal bone and viscera from the sacs, being careful not to break any black-containing sacs. Remove the tentacles and keep them aside. Mix the catalonia, ricotta, 3/4 sprigs of chopped marjoram, breadcrumbs and a pinch of salt and pepper in a bowl. Place the filling in a pastry bag and fill the calamari. Close your mouth with a toothpick. Cook the squid and tentacles for 5 minutes in a hot pan with a drizzle of oil. Season with salt. Served with vegetables of your choice.

COD IN TEMPURA WITH LIVORNESE SAUCE AND GREEN BEANS

Time 40 min

ingredients

4 people

For the cod

720 g 4 slices of desalted and soaked cod

100 g of flour 0, 100 g of corn starch

sparkling water

peanut oil, for the sauce

500 g of datterini cherry tomatoes

400 g of boiled green beans

200 g of dried tomatoes

20 g of desalted capers

4 spring onions, 1 clove of garlic

extra virgin olive oil, salt and pepper

Preparation

For the cod, mix the type 0 flour and the cornstarch with 200 g of sparkling water. Dip the cod steaks in the batter obtained, drain them and fry them in plenty of peanut oil at 170°C for at least 5/6 minutes. Place them on kitchen paper. For the sauce Soak the dried tomatoes for about ten minutes, then drain them and chop them finely with a knife. Sauté the spring onions in 3/4 tablespoons of oil, then add the blended datterini tomatoes and cook over medium heat for 58 minutes; add the dried tomatoes and continue for 23 minutes, season with salt and pepper and turn off. Fry the green beans in a pan with 2 tablespoons of oil, the garlic and capers. Serve the tempura cod with the sauce and green beans, garnished with fresh aromatic herbs if desired.

MUSHROOMS IN PAPER WITH CRISPY POLENTA

Time 1h

ingredients

4 people

For the polenta

200 g of coveted corn flour

125 g of boiled red beans

125 g of boiled borlotti beans

thyme, rosemary

fennel seeds

extra virgin olive oil

garlic, salt, for the mushrooms

1 kg of cardoncelli mushrooms

10 bay leaves, 1 head of garlic

Rosemary, sage, salt

white pepper, cloves

Juniper berries

Cinnamon sticks

extra virgin olive oil

Preparation

For the polenta, bring 1 liter of water to the boil with 1 tablespoon of oil and 1 teaspoon of salt; then pour in the flour and cook over a low heat, stirring constantly, for about 40 minutes. Chop 1 teaspoon of fennel seeds with a clove of garlic, a few sage leaves, a few rosemary leaves and thyme.

Mix the polenta with the chopped herbs and beans. Spread the polenta into a plumcake mold lined with cling film and leave to cool. Unmold the polenta, now cold and firm, cut it into slices and toast it in a pan with a drizzle of herb oil until the slices are crispy. For the mushrooms, prepare a parcel: spread a large sheet of aluminum foil on a plate, cover it with a bed of rosemary, sage and bay leaves, add 1 head of garlic cut in half lengthwise and arrange the mushrooms cut in half lengthwise long; season with extra virgin olive oil, salt, peppercorns, a few cloves, a piece of cinnamon and a few juniper berries. Partially close the foil to let the steam escape and bake at 250°C for 10/13 minutes. Serve the mushrooms with the polenta.

CHICKEN ROLL WITH CHESTNUT

Time 1h 50min

ingredients

Servings for 6 people

1.7 kg 1 headless chicken, cleaned

700 g of chestnuts

thyme, butter

extra virgin olive oil

salt, pepper, bay leaf

Preparation

For the chestnut chicken roll recipe, cook the chestnuts in boiling water with 1 bay leaf for about 40 minutes. Drain them with a slotted spoon and peel them. Remove the chicken at the end of the wings, then debone the dirt by cutting from the back: you will have to open it and "slide" the bones until obtain a layer of pulp lying on the skin. Pound the chicken with the meat tenderizer to get an even layer. Then place it on a sheet of baking paper, skin side down. Season with salt and pepper, flavor with thyme leaves, then fill the central part with chestnuts. Wrap the chicken in paper, closing the roll at the ends, then tie it with kitchen string and place it on a baking tray. Drizzle everything with a drizzle of oil and bake at 180°C for 15 minutes. Wet the pan with a ladle of the chestnut cooking water and cook for another 50 minutes. Remove from the oven and remove the roll from the pan. Wet all the scraps with a ladle of the chestnut cooking water and put the pan back in the oven for 5 minutes, so that the hot water dissolves all the caramelized crusts. Filter the tasty broth obtained into a saucepan, reduce it slightly on the heat, then add 20 g of butter, thus obtaining a sauce.

KOFTA (MIDDLE EASTERN MEATBALLS)

Time 40 minutes

ingredients

4 people

500 g finely minced meat

160 g of low-fat yogurt

120 g of tomato puree, 100 g of onion

4 cardamom pods

4 cloves, 3 cloves of garlic

1 cinnamon stick

red chilli powder, turmeric powder

fresh ginger, asafoetida

chickpea flour, salt

extra virgin olive oil

Preparation

For the kofta (Middle Eastern meatballs) recipe, sear the minced meat in a pan with a few tablespoons of water for 1 minute, then remove the water, draining the meat well. Put the meat back in the pan and cook for a couple of minutes; discard the liquid it has released again. Add 2 tablespoons of yogurt, 1 teaspoon of red chili powder, 1 tablespoon of grated ginger, a good pinch of asafoetida, 2 cloves of garlic previously pureed, 50 g of chopped onion and 2 tablespoons of chickpea flour. Mix everything and add salt. Form meatballs the size of a ping pong ball, possibly adding more chickpea flour to give the right consistency.

Dredge the meatballs in chickpea flour. Heat a few tablespoons of extra virgin olive oil in a shallow pan and brown the meatballs for about 5 minutes, until they are golden. Heat 50 g of mustard or extra virgin olive oil in a pan, add the cinnamon, cloves, cardamom pods and a good pinch of asafoetida. When the spices start to sizzle, add 50g of chopped onion and continue cooking until the onion has turned pink. Add 1 tablespoon of grated ginger, the garlic clove previously pureed and ½ teaspoon of turmeric; lower the heat, leave to infuse for 1 minute, then add the tomato puree and the remaining yogurt, continuing to cook over low heat, stirring, for 45 minutes. Add the meatballs and continue cooking for another 56 minutes. Serve them as desired with bean sprouts, salad, rice or crusty bread.

PRAWNS, CHICKPEAS E CHICKPEAS WITH FOAM

Time 40 min

ingredients

Portions for 4 people

50 g of pomegranate seeds

50 g boiled canned chickpeas

16 g of prawns

2 heads of long red radicchio

sugar, white vinegar, bay leaf

extra virgin olive oil, salt and pepper

Preparation

For the recipe of prawns, radicchio and chickpeas with foam, add the chickpeas and mash them with 1 bay leaf for 10 minutes.

Turn off and let the chickpeas cool in their water. Cut the radicchio heads into 6 segments each and brown them in a pan with a drizzle of oil, salt and pepper. Cut the prawns in half lengthwise, without shelling them. Roast in a pan with a drizzle of oil and a pinch of salt, placing first on the meat side for 2 minutes, then on the shells for 1/2 minute. Remove them from the pan, and toast the pomegranate seeds in the same pan for 1 minute with a pinch of sugar and a pinch of salt, then add 3 tablespoons of white vinegar. Drain the chickpeas, reserving the cooking water. Season the chickpeas with a drizzle of oil and, if needed, salt. Weigh 180 g of the chickpea cooking water and whip them with a whisk, like an egg white, until you obtain a firm foam. Serve the prawns with radicchio and chickpeas,

LIVER, ONIONS, AND APPLES

Time 40 min

ingredients

Portions for 4 people

450 g 4 slices of veal liver

3 white onions

2 green Golden apples

bay flour

dry white wine

extra virgin olive oil

butter, salt, pepper

Preparation

For the liver, onions and apples recipe, cut the liver into strips. Finely slice the onions. Wash the apples and, without peeling them, cut them into pieces. Heat a drizzle of oil in a pan, add the apples and onions, season them with salt, pepper and 2 bay leaves and cook for about 15 minutes; then blend with the white wine and continue until the onion has become transparent and very tender. Free the pan and melt a knob of butter on the same bottom; add the liver, dusted with a little flour, salt and pepper; add a splash of white wine and cook by sautéing for a couple of minutes. Serve immediately with a side dish of apples and onions.

AROMATIC MUSSELS WITH FRENCH FRIES AND TWO MAYONNAISE

Time 40 minutes

ingredients

4 people

2 kg of mussels

1.5 kg of potatoes

300 g of mayonnaise

150g of red chilli pepper

2 celery hearts

1 onion, garlic, thyme

mustard, parsley, pepper

dry white wine

extra virgin olive oil

Preparation

For the recipe of aromatic mussels with french fries and two mayonnaise, peel the potatoes and cut them into sticks. Rinse under water, in a bowl, until the water runs clear. Dry them well with kitchen paper and fry them in plenty of peanut oil, at 160°C, for about 8/10 minutes: with this first cooking the potatoes soften and cook well inside. Drain them on kitchen paper and keep the oil hot. Clean the mussels and rinse. Peel and chop the onion, celery and pepper. Prepare a bunch with thyme and parsley, tying it with kitchen twine. Heat a drizzle of extra virgin olive oil in a saucepan, add the chopped vegetables and let them sweat for 2 minutes.

Add the mussels and the bouquet garni, mix, pepper and deglaze with 1/2 glass of wine. Cover with a lid and cook for about 2 minutes, until the mussels have opened. Fry the chips again, at 190°C, to brown them and create a crunchy crust on the outside. Mix half the mayonnaise with 1 teaspoon mustard. Mix the remaining mayonnaise with 1/2 clove of squeezed garlic and 1 tablespoon of chopped parsley. Serve the mussels with the chips, accompanied by the two mayonnaises.

MEDITERRANEAN-STYLE COD IN AGUACHILE

Time 20 min

ingredients

4 people

600 g of skinless cod fillet

15 g of desalted capers

10 grams of fresh coriander

5 g of fresh parsley

1 serrano type of green chili pepper

1 lime, 1 lemon

extra virgin olive oil

salt and pepper

Preparation

For the recipe for Mediterranean cod in aguanile, prepare the agua chile sauce: blend the coriander and parsley leaves (keep some whole to complete) with the lime juice and 1/2 lemon, a pinch of salt, 2 tablespoons of oil and green chili pepper. Grease a non-stick pan with a drizzle of oil, drain the cod over high heat for 23 minutes per side, then lightly salt, close with the lid and continue over low heat for another 56 minutes. Distribute the cod onto plates, complete with 1 tablespoon of capers, the aguachile sauce and, to taste, lemon or lime wedges. Top with parsley or coriander leaves. The ingredient: Serrano chili pepper is a whole green chili pepper native to Mexico. If not too spicy, it can be replaced with other similar varieties.

PORK FILLET WITH LIEGE SYRUP, FRIGGITELLI AND SPILLION ONIONS

Time 35 min

ingredients

4 people

500 g of peeled Borettane onions

600 g 1 piece of pork fillet

400 g of friggitelli peppers

thyme, bay leaf

extra virgin olive oil

salt and pepper

Preparation

For the recipe of pork fillet with Liège syrup, friggitelli and spring onions, salt and pepper the fillet, sprinkle with chopped thyme and brown it on all sides in a pan with a drizzle of oil, for about 6/7 minutes. Add the spring onions, a couple of bay leaves, 2 tablespoons of Liège syrup, salt and pepper and cook until the fillet reaches 58°C in the centre, about 20 minutes, turning several times. During cooking the onions will release a little water, which will serve to dilute the syrup and meat juices, creating a sauce. Check evaporation during cooking and, if necessary, add a drop of water. Separately, sauté the friggitelli in another pan with a drizzle of oil for 8/10 minutes. Serve the roast with its sauce and onions; completed with friggitelli, the Mediterranean note in a more continental dish.

SEABASS WITH INDIAN SPICES (TAKA TAK)

Time 30 min + 1h rest

ingredients

4 people

4 sea bass fillets

For the marinade

yogurt, turmeric

carom seeds

red chilli powder

fresh ginger, honey

lime juice

extra virgin olive oil

salt, black pepper

For the sauce

butter, salt

carom seeds

lime juice, saffron

Preparation

For the Marinade Toast 1 teaspoon of carom seeds, ½ teaspoon of black pepper and ½ teaspoon of chili pepper in a pan for about 3 minutes, until you can smell it. Pulverize the spices in a mortar, then add 1 teaspoon of chopped ginger and continue to crush; finally add 2 tablespoons of yogurt, 1 teaspoon of honey, a pinch of salt, 1 teaspoon of lime juice, 1 teaspoon of turmeric and 3 tablespoons of oil, mixing well. Pour the mixture over the fish fillets and place in the refrigerator for 1 hour.

Oil a flat pan and grill the fish for about 2 minutes per side. For the sauce, heat 2 tablespoons butter, add 1/2 tablespoon carom seeds, 1/2 tablespoon lime juice, and 1 tablespoon water; reduce for 1 minute, add salt, then add 23 saffron threads, previously rehydrated in warm water, and reduce for a further couple of minutes. Arrange the fish on plates, sprinkle it with the sauce and complete it to taste with flowers, aromatic herbs and plenty of turmeric powder.

BREAM AND CARAMELIZED ENDIVE

Time 1h

ingredients

Portions for 4 people

2 sea bream, 800 g each.

4 heads of Belgian endive

honey, lemon, garlic

sage, rosemary

thyme, bay leaf

Dry Marsala, butter

extra virgin olive oil

salt and pepper

Preparation

For the sea bream and caramelized endive recipe, clean the sea bream: scale them, cut the fins and gut them; obtain 4 fillets, trimming the ventral part, which is softer and full of bones. Keep the head, midbone and belly cutouts. Brown all the fish scraps in a pan with a thin layer of oil, a sprig of rosemary, a little thyme and 1 bay leaf; after 10/15 minutes add 1/2 glass of dry Marsala, and continue cooking for another 30 minutes, stirring occasionally; finally filter and thicken the sauce on the heat, with a small piece of butter, for 5 minutes.

In a pan, heat a drizzle of oil with a sprig of rosemary, 2 sage leaves and 1 clove of garlic over medium heat; add the sea bream fillets, placing them skin side down, cover with the lid and cook for about ten minutes. Cut the 4 endive heads in half and steam for 10 minutes. In the meantime, blend 3 tablespoons of honey with 3 tablespoons of oil and 2 lemon peels, salt and pepper and, to taste, a few chervil leaves. Transfer the endive to a baking tray, brush with the honey emulsion and bake at 200°C for 45 minutes. Serve the sea bream fillets with the sauce and accompany them with the escarole.

MARENGO CHICKEN

Time 45 min

ingredients

Servings for 6 people

1.2kg 1 chicken

500 grams of tomatoes

150 g clean

Champignon mushrooms

6 eggs,

6 prawn tails

flour, garlic, lemon

homemade bread

butter, salt

chopped parsley, dry white wine

extra virgin olive oil

Preparation

For the chicken Marengo recipe, cut the chicken into 6 pieces, separating the breast and thighs. Flour them and brown them in a large pan with a drizzle of oil, a knob of butter and 1 clove of garlic crushed in its peel. Turn the pieces on all sides for 5/6 minutes. Deglaze the chicken with 1 glass of wine, then add the chopped tomatoes. Add salt and cook for 5 minutes. Remove the breasts and add the sliced mushrooms. Cook for another 10 minutes, then add the breasts again, the juice of 1/2 lemon and 2 tablespoons of parsley and finish cooking in 12 minutes. Toast 6 slices of bread. Fry the fried eggs for 5 minutes. Roast the shelled prawn tails, then add them to the sauce with the chicken. Serve the chicken in its sauce, with the egg on the bread.

BAKED MULLET WITH YOGURT FUMETTO

Time 45 min

ingredients

2 people

700 g 6 red mullets

100 g of natural whole yoghurt

10 datterini tomatoes

2 cloves of garlic

1 shallot, 1 onion

1 fennel, lemon

extra virgin olive oil

Chia seeds

dry white wine

salt and pepper

Preparation

For the recipe for baked mullet with yogurt fumet, clean the mullet and open them like a book, holding them together by the tail. Keep all scraps. Heat a drizzle of oil in a saucepan, add the red mullet scraps, the tomatoes, the garlic, the shallot and the peeled onion, the fennel stems and the barbine. Add 100 g of white wine and 1/2 liter of water; let it simmer on a low heat for about twenty minutes, then filter and reduce the resulting broth, always over low heat, for 1015 minutes, so that the flavors concentrate. In the meantime, place the red mullets on a baking tray lined with baking paper, season them with a drizzle of oil, salt, pepper and grated lemon zest and bake at 200°C for about 10 minutes. Mix the fumet with the yogurt to obtain a sauce. Cut the fennel very thin and season it with oil, salt and lemon.

SWEET AND SOUR RABBIT

Time 1h

ingredients

4 people

1.5 kg 1 rabbit

300 g of aubergines, 60 g of honey

2 stalks of celery

1 onion, green olives

salted capers, parsley

white almonds

extra virgin olive oil

salt, pepper, vinegar

Preparation

For the sweet and sour rabbit recipe, clean
the rabbit, remove its entrails and cut it

in chunks. Brown in a large rondo with 4
tablespoons of oil, roasting on all sides for
about 10 minutes, adding salt and pepper.
Stone about 20 olives. Clean the celery stalks
and cut them into small pieces; peel the
onion and slice it. Rinse 1 tablespoon of
capers from salt. Mix olives, celery, onion
and capers and season with salt and pepper.
Deglaze the cooking rabbit with 130 g of
vinegar and add the honey. Cook for 2
minutes, then add the mixed vegetables.
Cover, reduce the heat and cook for about 10
minutes. Peel the aubergine and cut it into
small pieces. Cook it in a pan with 4/5
tablespoons of oil for about 10 minutes, until
it browns. Finally, add the aubergines to the
rabbit and cook for another 10 minutes,
turning the pieces of meat from time to time.
Turn off and let cool. Serve the rabbit with
the vegetables, complete with chopped
parsley and chopped almonds.

SHELL SOUP

Time 1h + 12h rest

ingredients

4 people

800 g of mussels

400 g of homemade bread

300 g clams

300 g sea truffles

200 g of yellow cherry tomatoes

200 g of red cherry tomatoes

1 clove of garlic

parsley

lemon, white wine

extra virgin olive oil

salt fine and coarse

Preparation

For the conch soup recipe, soak the clams and sea truffles in separate bowls. Let them drain for 12 hours, changing the water often. Brush the sea truffles, which often accumulate sand even on the outside. Rinse the mussels under water, then remove the filament and, to remove it completely, pull it towards the rounded base of the shell. Then collect them in a bowl with 2 handfuls of coarse salt and rubbed together, to clean the shells well, finally rinse under water. Cut the red cherry tomatoes in half and place them in the pan with a drizzle of oil, 1 clove of garlic and 2 stalks of parsley.

After 2 minutes add the clams, cover them
and let them open for 2 minutes. Cut the
yellow tomatoes in half and place them in a
saucepan with a drizzle of oil. Add the
truffles, add a drop of wine, cover and let
them open for 23 minutes. Open the mussels
in a saucepan with a lid for 12 minutes. Filter
the water from the mussels and truffles and
save it for the soup. Combine all the other
shells and yellow tomatoes in the pan with
the clams. Complete with 1 ladle of filtered
water and mix everything together. Spread
them on slices of toasted bread and complete
the soup with parsley leaves and grated
lemon zest.

SALT CRUSTED SEABASS WITH ORANGE SALAD

Time 35 min

ingredients

4 people

400 g 4 slices of sea bass fillet

400 g of whole sea salt

80 g of egg white

2 spring onions

2 medium fennel hearts

1 orange

pitted black olives

extra virgin olive oil

salt and pepper

Preparation

For the recipe for sea bass in a salt crust with orange salad, whip the egg white until stiff and mix it with the brown salt. Line a pan with aluminum foil, pour in the salted meringue and place it on the heat. When the meringue is hot, place the sea bass slices skin side down. Cover with another sheet of aluminum foil and cook the fish gently for about 15 minutes. Peel the orange (eliminating all the skins); remove the segments and cut them into small pieces. Mix them with the sliced spring onions, thinly sliced fennel and pitted olives. Season with oil, salt and pepper. Distribute the salad on plates, arrange the sea bass fillets, finish with a drizzle of oil and serve.

POTATO OMELETTES

Time 20 min

ingredients

Portions for 4 people

500 g of yellow-fleshed potatoes

2 egg whites

extra virgin olive oil

salt

Preparation

For the potato omelette recipe, peel and grate the potatoes with a grater with large holes; squeeze them and dry them with a cloth. Mix the potatoes with the lightly beaten egg whites and a pinch of salt. Heat a non-stick pan with a thin layer of oil, pour in the egg white and potato mixture and mix lightly. As soon as it starts to brown, wrap it up giving it the shape of an omelette.

SPOON PUMPKIN

Time 1h

ingredients

4 servings

1 butternut squash

50 g of peeled pumpkin seeds

1 pc shallot

vegetable broth

Pepper

salt

extra virgin olive oil

sugar

Preparation

For the spoonful pumpkin recipe, choose a long pumpkin and cut it into three parts, obtaining the round part at the base, the long one in the center, and the cap.

Scoop out the rounded part with a spoon. Season it inside with a drizzle of oil, salt and pepper. Place on a plate together with the shell (if you want you can use it as a lid) and bake at 200°C for 40 minutes. Peel the elongated part and cut the pulp into cubes. Slice the shallot and fry it in a pan with a drizzle of oil; add the pumpkin cut into cubes, add 2 ladles of broth and cook over low heat for about 20 minutes, adding more broth as it dries. Cook 2 tablespoons of sugar in a pan with 2 tablespoons of water and a pinch of salt. When the sugar has dissolved, add the pumpkin seeds and mix until the sugar sticks to the seeds, «rewarding». Turn it off and let it cool. Remove the pumpkin from the oven, fill it with the cubes cooked in the pan and complete it with the crunchy seeds.

SEARED TUNA WITH BROWNED AND FRIED ONIONS

Time 35 min

ingredients

Portions for 4 people

900 g of fresh tuna fillet

500 grams of onions

extra virgin olive oil

salt

Pepper

Preparation

For the seared tuna with browned and fried onions recipe, immerse the tuna in a pot full of boiling salted water for a couple of minutes. Drain it and let it cool. Cut the onions into very thin slices. Brown 300 g in a drizzle of oil, sprinkle them with a drop of water, add salt and stew for about 20 minutes. Then blend them with the immersion blender, obtaining a sauce. Fry the remaining onions in boiling oil and drain them on kitchen paper. Cut the tuna into slices and serve it with the fried and blended onions, complete with salt and pepper.

PORK LOIN WITH PECORINO SAUCE

Time 35 min

ingredients

Portions for 4 people

400g sliced pork loin

200 g of milk

150 g of pecorino

2 g of corn starch

garlic

parsley, fennel

fresh oregano

sage, salt

extra virgin olive oil

Preparation

For the pork loin with pecorino sauce recipe, clean the pork loin slices and sprinkle with salt. Prepare the finely chopped parsley, fennel and oregano. Roast the meat in a pan covered with oil on both sides with 1 unpeeled clove of garlic and a few sage leaves. Finally, season with the chopped aromatic herbs. Dissolve the cornstarch in 2 tablespoons of cold water. Bring the milk to the boil, dissolve the dissolved cornstarch in it and stir until it begins to thicken. Remove from the heat and add the grated pecorino. Distribute the pecorino sauce on the plates, arrange the chops and complete with other aromatic herbs as desired.

**CHICKEN BITES
WITH TOMATO AND
ONIONS VELVETE**

Time 45 min

ingredients

Portions for 4 people

1 chicken

150 g of tomato puree

1 onion

1 clove of garlic

dry white wine

extra virgin olive oil

Rosemary

salt and pepper

Preparation

For the recipe for chicken nuggets with tomato and onion cream, divide the chicken into pieces and debone. Cut the pulp into small pieces. Brown the meat in a pan with a drizzle of oil, the crushed garlic clove and a sprig of rosemary. Deglaze with a splash of white wine, add the tomato puree, salt and pepper and cook for another 15 minutes. Remove the meat and keep it aside. Remove the garlic and rosemary, then blend the cooking liquid until you obtain a velvety sauce. Clean the onion and peel it, separating the skins. Brown for 5 minutes in a pan with a drizzle of oil, salt and rosemary. Serve the chicken with the sauce and onion.

SWEET AND SOUR TROUT

Time 25 min

ingredients

Servings for 24 people

2 salmon trout fillets

300 g of green beans

1 pink grapefruit

already pitted green olives

1 red onion

vinegar

White wine

extra virgin olive oil

salt, peppercorns

Preparation

For the sweet and sour trout recipe, clean the green beans, boil them for 67 minutes in boiling salted water and drain them. Slice the onion and sauté it with 50 g of vinegar, 50 g of wine and a little pepper for 3 minutes after boiling. Divide the grapefruit into segments and, if you want, remove the peel. Drain the onion, reserving the cooking liquid. Arrange the trout fillets on plates with the green beans, onion, olives and grapefruit. Season them with the oil and the onion liquid.

FRESH LIGURIAN FISH BURRIDA

Time 1h 35min

ingredients

Serves 8 people

850 g 1 gurnard

700 g croaker

680 g 8 slices of monkfish

600 g of tomatoes, 300 g of calamari

250 g of baby octopus

150 grams of onion

16 small red prawns

8 scampi, 8 cuttlefish

extra virgin olive oil

dry white wine

dried oregano

salt and pepper

Preparation

For the Ligurian recipe for fresh fish burrida, clean and fillet gurnard and croaker, then peel the fillets and cut them into chunks. Cut the monkfish into slices. Clean the octopus, squid and cuttlefish. Blanch the tomatoes in boiling water, remove the skin and seeds and cut the fillets into cubes. Slice the onion. Assemble the casserole: distribute half the onion and tomatoes on the bottom, greased with a drizzle of oil; add the fish steaks, then the crustaceans and molluscs; cover the fish with the remaining onion and tomato. Pour in 2 glasses of wine, flavor with oil, dried oregano, salt and pepper and cook for approximately 1 hour and 30 minutes.

PIZZA STEAKS

Time 25 min

ingredients

Portions for 4 people

200 g of tomato puree

400 g slices of rump

of beef 100 g each.

extra virgin olive oil

dried oregano

1 clove of garlic

salt

Pepper

Preparation

For the pizzaiola steak recipe, lightly beat the rump slices until they are 4/5 mm thick. Heat gently in a pan, without frying, 2 tablespoons of oil with the sliced garlic. Add the tomato puree, cook for about ten minutes, and season with salt, pepper and a little dried oregano. Add the slices of meat to the sauce and cook them for 3 minutes; turn them and cook for another 4/5 minutes, depending on the thickness. Serve them with the sauce and oregano.

CHICKEN PEACH AND GREEN BEAN SALAD,

Time 1h 20min

ingredients

6 people

900 g 3 chicken legs with thighs

200 g of iceberg lettuce

150 g of cucumbers

100 g of green beans

50 g of tuna in oil

3 peaches, 1 onion

1 carrot, 1 celery stalk

dry white wine

bay leaf, parsley

vinegar, spring onion

extra virgin olive oil

coarse salt and peppercorns

Preparation

For the chicken, peach and green bean salad recipe, prepare an aromatic broth with the onion, the celery stalk, the carrot, 1 glass of white wine, a few peppercorns, 1 bay leaf, 2 sprigs of parsley and a a handful of coarse salt; when it boils, add the chicken and cook for 35 minutes. Turn off the heat and let the chicken cool in the cooking broth. Peel the striped cucumber, remove the central seeds, cut it into thin slices and marinate it in 4 tablespoons of vinegar for 30 minutes, stirring occasionally, then squeeze it well. Peel the green beans and cook them in boiling water for about 8 minutes.

Drain E, cool them under running water and, if you like, divide them in half lengthwise. Cut the iceberg lettuce into strips and wash them well. Finely slice 10 g of the white part of the spring onion. Remove the bones and skin from the chicken and shred the meat. Add the well-drained tuna, the spring onion, the marinated cucumber, the peaches cut into segments with the skin, 4 tablespoons of oil, a good pinch of salt and mix well. Arrange the iceberg lettuce strips on the plates, complete with the seasoned chicken and serve.

STUFFED ARTICHOKES NEAPOLITAN STYLE

Time 40 min

ingredients

Servings for 46 people

250 g of boiled beef

60 g grated parmesan

50 g of tomato sauce

30 g of onion

30 g of breadcrumbs

10 artichokes, 1 egg

parsley, lemon

dry white wine

extra virgin olive oil

salt and pepper

Preparation

For the Neapolitan-style stuffed artichokes recipe, peel the artichokes, removing the stem and outer leaves. Remove the internal beard, using a perforator. Place them, as they are cleaned, in a basin of water with the juice of 1/2 lemon. Boil them in boiling water acidulated with lemon juice for 10 minutes. Chop the onion and fry it in a saucepan in a drizzle of oil with the boiled meat for a couple of minutes. Add the tomato sauce and cook for another 5 minutes. Turn off, let cool, then chop everything; mix with a sprig of chopped parsley, the parmesan and the egg and season with salt and pepper. Stuff the emptied artichokes with this filling and arrange in a baking dish. Pour 1/2 glass of wine on the bottom and sprinkle the artichokes with breadcrumbs, grease with a drizzle of oil and bake at 180°C for about 15 minutes.

TUNA WITH ONIONS, THE SARDINIAN RECIPE

Time 40 min

ingredients

Portions for 4 people

700 g tuna steak

250 g of red onion

extra virgin olive oil

salt

Preparation

For the Sardinian tuna with onions recipe, place the tuna in a saucepan full of water. Add salt and bring to the boil, then cook for 30 minutes. Peel the onion and slice. Place it in a bowl immersed in hot water, so that it loses its acidity. Let it rest for 10 minutes. Drain the tuna and serve hot with the onion and a drizzle of oil.

GRILLED SALMON WITH MUSTARD AND HONEY SAUCE

Preparation time: 15 minutes

Cooking time: 15 minutes

Doses for 2 people:

Ingredients:

2 salmon fillets

2 tablespoons of mustard

1 tablespoon honey

1 tablespoon of oil

extra virgin olive oil

Salt and Pepper To Taste

Preparation:

Preheat grill to medium-high heat. In a bowl, mix the mustard, honey, extra virgin olive oil, salt and pepper. Brush the salmon fillets with the mixture obtained. Grill salmon for 57 minutes per side, or until cooked through. Serve the grilled salmon with mustard sauce and hot honey.

CONCLUSION

Thank you for embarking on this journey to better health with "Insulin Resistance Diet 2025". We hope that the information, nutritional strategies, and meal plans presented in this book have given you the tools you need to manage insulin resistance effectively. Our goal was to offer you a complete guide based on scientific evidence, capable of improving your quality of life and preventing complications related to this condition. An Invitation to Leave a Review Your feedback is extremely important to us. If you found this book useful, we kindly invite you to leave a review.

Your opinions not only help us improve, but also provide valuable information to other readers who could benefit from this knowledge. An honest, detailed review can make a difference and help other people find the support they need to manage insulin resistance. Thank you again for your time and effort in reading "Insulin Resistance Diet 2025". We wish you success in your health and wellness journey. With gratitude,

[KLARLOCK]

www.ingramcontent.com/pod-product-compliance
Lightning Source LLC
Chambersburg PA
CBHW070651250726
48662CB00001B/65